INFERTILITY IN THE BIBLE

HOW THE MATRIARCHS CHANGED THEIR FATE

HOW YOU CAN TOO

By Jessie Fischbein

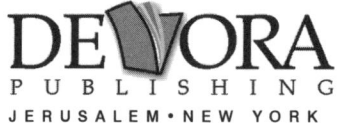

PUBLISHING

JERUSALEM • NEW YORK

INFERTILITY IN THE BIBLE:
How the Matriarchs Changed Their Fate, How You Can Too

Published by DEVORA PUBLISHING COMPANY

Text Copyright © 2005 by Jessie Fischbein
Editor: Fern Levitt
Cover and Book Design: Benjie Herskowitz

Credits: Rabbi Joseph B, Soloveitchik, FATE AND DESTINY: FROM HOLOCAUST TO THE STATE OF ISRAEL. Ktav Publishing House, Hoboken, New Jersey, 1992, 2000
Nechama Leibowitz, STUDIES IN BERESHIT. Printed by the publishing dept. of the Jewish Agency, Jerusalem, Israel, 1976

All rights reserved. No part of this book may be reproduced or transmitted in any form or by any means, electronic or mechanical, including photocopying, recording, or by any information storage and retrieval system, without permission in writing from the publisher.

Hard Cover ISBN: 1-932687-34-3
Soft Cover ISBN: 1-932687-35-1

Email: sales@devorapublishing.com
Web Site: www.devorapublishing.com

Printed in Israel

For you. And for me.

Acknowledgements

Thank you, Emily Amie Witty. Without you, this book would still be an outline.

Thank you, Rivki Khesin, who held my hand through every chapter and taught me what it means for a book to be readable.

Thank you to Rabbi Reuven Mann and my other Rebbes, who have revealed to me how the Torah is a tree of life for those who grab onto it.

Thank you to my editor, Fern Levitt, for your skill, dexterity with language, and enthusiasm.

Thanks to my parents for their love and support.

And thanks most of all to my husband Ari, whose wisdom and clarity have been my indispensable source of encouragement.

Jessie Fischbein
New York
February 2005

Table of Contents

Introduction		9
Chapter I.	**Premises**	13
Chapter II.	**How the Matriarchs Coped with Infertility**	26
Chapter III.	**Sarah**	37
Chapter IV.	**The Journey and Divine Intervention**	55
Chapter V.	**Rebecca**	72
Chapter VI.	**Rachel**	81
Chapter VII.	**The Real Purpose of Your Existence**	90
Chapter VIII.	**Rachel Continued**	93
Chapter IX.	**Leah and Rachel's Sibling Rivalry**	107
Chapter X.	**The Matriarchs' Stories:**	
	What Does It All Mean?	115
Chapter XI.	**Michal**	130
Chapter XII.	**Hannah**	133
Chapter XIII.	**The Power of Prayer**	149
Chapter XIV.	**Hannah Continued**	157
Chapter XV.	**How Does Prayer Work?**	162
Chapter XVI.	**When Prayer Isn't Answered**	171
Chapter XVII.	**King David and Infant Loss**	176
Chapter XVIII.	**Final Thoughts**	184
Meet the Commentators		187
Bibliography		191

Introduction

I have been thinking about how to start this book for a long time. In fact, I've been thinking about this entire book for a long time. I wanted to begin with a paragraph that adequately describes the sharp pang that an infertile woman experiences as she sees a pregnant woman walk past, or a woman pushing a stroller. As opposed to the dull, throbbing pain she feels as she goes about her daily activities, trying to live a life that feels in some ways purposeless. As opposed to the sinking despair as she sees the blood of her period. Another month gone.

Then there's the isolation when you are in social situations with your peers and they chat about their children. The anger at people's insensitivity. And many other subtle and not-so-subtle pains.

If pain was one-dimensional, we might cope with it better. As it is, our infertility interacts with the situations we encounter and triggers many different types of suffering and pain.

Many people look to the Bible for inspiration in times of suffering. It may seem ironic that most people turn to religious inspiration only when pain hits, but it actually makes a lot of sense. Most people are content to operate within the laws of nature, and rightly so. After all, modern scientists have ably demonstrated the notion of cause and effect, action and consequence.

But what happens when the laws of nature aren't satisfactory? When circumstance painfully knocks you over? Humans seek other explanations. Our hearts conjure up a Being, One Who is In Control, who must be doing this to us. Fear and insecurity are the prime motivations for Man seeking God.

If you are in this state, and you are interested in what the Bible has to say about infertility (and it does have plenty to say on the subject), this book was designed to guide you on your tour.

I have chosen to address infertile women directly throughout the book because I feel that this lets me have a personal, intimate conversation with the reader. I know that this is not the profile of every reader, but I hope that others who may read the book – husbands, other family members, counseling professionals – may identify and in that way deepen their own understanding of the issue by imagining themselves in the position of a woman experiencing infertility.

When I personally encountered difficulty in conceiving, I researched the possible medical causes of infertility and the available medical treatments. But nowhere was I able to find a book that dealt with the spiritual aspect of infertility. What is the response to infertility as it affects my relationship with the Creator? What are the spiritual causes and the spiritual treatments?

Of course, the Bible discusses all of that. But sometimes it's helpful to have a tour guide.

As I delved into the subject, I found it comforting to know that I was not alone; in fact, I was in good company. Our most important female role models, the Matriarchs, experienced the pain of infertility, as do one in ten modern American couples (approximately 6.1 million couples, according to a Google search I performed in 2001) who have difficulty in conceiving without intervention. The Bible maintains that a Creator directs the physical universe and the laws of nature. So I wondered how this widespread phenomenon relates to the Creator.

This book is my attempt to share the avenues I explored as I thought and studied about this question. Writing it has been a profound experience for me and I hope and believe that you will find reading it a gateway to growth. I cannot guarantee that you will no longer feel pangs of desire mingled with sadness at the sight of a pregnant woman or sounds of children laughing. But I hope that, after reading this book, you will have a changed perspective... when you look at you.

> *Note:* Some of the premises may strike you as self-explanatory; I included them because they are the foundation of everything I am saying.

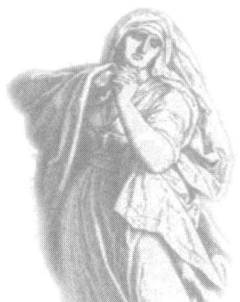

Chapter I
Premises

The Bible is generally acknowledged to be a book of inspiration. If you don't agree, don't let it stop you from reading further. This is actually *not* one of my premises. I consider it my obligation to demonstrate that the Bible is meaningful.

Before we begin our investigation of infertility in the Bible, I will set forth my premises so you'll know up front where you may vehemently disagree with me. I'm sure we'll manage to find some common ground.

Why do you need to know my premises? To paraphrase Maimonides, a Middle Ages[1] scholar: "Know, my masters, that you should not believe anything unless you can see/touch/hear it; you can logically prove it, or someone you trust[2] said it."[3]

All things that are reasonable to believe fit into one of these three categories. Maimonides recommends that we examine our doctrinal beliefs (the things we accept as true) and figure out which of those three reasons explains why we believe it. If we can't fit it into one of those categories, and we still think it's reasonable to believe, it's probably worth further thought.

He adds a friendly warning that might make us think twice before we accept doctrinal beliefs: "One, however, who bases his belief on anything except for these three sources, Scriptures refers to him as 'the fool believes everything." (Proverbs 14:15.)

Premises

First things first. I am an Orthodox Jew. What that means to me is that I consider myself obligated to keep the laws given in the Bible, which I call the *Torah* (from the Hebrew root *to teach*). I maintain that there is a group of people in existence today, the Jews, who are obligated to follow *all* of the laws set forth in the Torah (which others might call the Bible). I also maintain a set of fundamental principles which I'll share with you as they come up. The following are some of them:

The Bible

When I refer to the Bible or Torah, I am referring to the Five Books of Moses (Genesis, Exodus, Leviticus, Numbers, and Deuteronomy), the Prophets (Joshua, Judges, Samuel I and II, Kings I and II, Isaiah, Jeremiah, Ezekiel, and The Twelve Prophets), and the Writings (Psalms, Proverbs, Job, Song of Songs, Ruth, Lamentations or *Eicha* in Hebrew, Ecclesiastes or *Koheleth*, Esther, Daniel, Ezra-Nechemia, and Chronicles or *Divrei HaYamim*).

I have chosen passages that deal primarily and directly with the subject of infertility, largely from Genesis and the life stories of the Matriarchs Sarah, Rebecca (*Rivka*), Rachel and Leah, but have also included the stories of Michal from Samuel II and of Hannah (*Chana*) and her archrival Penina from Samuel I. On the related topic of loss of a baby, a chapter near the end of the book discusses King David's reaction to the death of his infant son.

Torah Is Divine

If you don't believe in God, or if you're not sure, or if you believe in a Creator but not in an Author, I'll be content with: "The Bible may or may not have something interesting to say about infertility that I can find useful." If you're willing to reserve judgment on that basis, we've got plenty to discuss.

The Five Books of Moses Were Given with a Divine Oral Explanation

That's right, while Moses was up on the mountain for forty days and forty nights (Exodus 24:18), God was teaching him the explanation of the Torah. This divine explanation was passed down orally until it was compiled, in two waves, one at around 200 A.D. (what we call the *Mishna*) and the other at around 500 A.D. (what we call the *Gemara*, or the Talmud).

Well, I can't talk you into accepting that. But how about this: Whenever you read a statement that I maintain is based on the Oral Law, you evaluate it on its own merit. If it makes sense to you, and you are able to gain some insight from it, then we'll work with that.

The Prerequisite of the Premise that Torah is Divine

Naturally, if I maintain that the Torah is divine, I maintain that the world exists as the result of a Creator's will. I also maintain that the Creator interacts with his creations. Giving us the Torah is one such interaction.

Now don't think if you're an atheist or an agnostic that we have nothing to work with. After all, doesn't AA have their "Higher Power" thing? And I'm sure there are recovering agnostic and atheist alcoholics.

Man's Unique Nature

Let's have a look at qualities that are unique to humans. You may think of some that I left out, but the ones that come to my mind are opposable thumbs, more sophisticated emotions than other animals, the capacity for self-reflection, and the ability to make "moral choices." (I know that last one's a fuzzy term that needs explanation.)

Actually, all of those (except for opposable thumbs, and according to some theories, even opposable thumbs) can be subsumed under the quality of "capable of abstract thought."

Some expansion on the idea of abstract thought and moral choices: a human being is unique in that his intellect can evaluate a situation and control his instincts if the evaluation calls for it, as opposed to an animal, which is caught in its instincts and has no other faculty. Although an animal has intelligence, his intelligence is in *service* of his instincts (a tiger intelligently figures out the best way to hunt its prey) and can never get beyond them.

This can be explained by one of my favorite examples: the deer in the headlights.

Scene one. A deer is peacefully chewing a plant in the forest. Suddenly, her ears perk up—danger! What does she do? She freezes. The instinct to freeze protects her beautifully. She blends into the forest, her camouflage rendering her invisible.

Scene two. A deer is peacefully standing on a road. Suddenly, a car comes zooming at her. The headlights catch her in their beams. What does she do? She freezes. The instinct to freeze that saved her in the forest now destroys her as she is unable to overcome her instinct—and the car crashes into her.

Scene three. A human being stands, petrified, as headlight beams come at him. He can't move. He's frozen. He has the same animal instinct of self-preservation as the deer. The car is coming closer. "Staying here is a bad idea," he thinks. "I have to move." But his body doesn't move by itself. Finally, with the force of his will, he overcomes his instinct and hurls himself out of the way. Mind overcomes instinct!

So what I'm saying is that the human mind, and how it relates to our instincts, is what makes us people unique.

Use the Same Standards of Reason to Decide on a Religious Tenet as to Make a Financial Decision

Nobody has to accept anything that doesn't make sense. Of course, the converse also applies—only accept what does make sense.

Strictly speaking, that is not a premise of Judaism, but is just the way our brains work. It seems obvious, so you might think I shouldn't even bother to state it. But I'm sure I'll be making recourse to this point.

A Note on How the Oral Law's Obscurity Leads to Clarity

As I have mentioned, the written Torah was given with an orally-passed-down counterpart. The Oral Law was compiled and written down by the sages of the Mishna and Talmud. We refer to them as *Chazal*, a term of respect that comes from the Hebrew acronym *Ch'Z'L* (*Chachameinu Zichronam Livracha*—Our Wise Ones of Blessed Memory). It is common practice to use the present tense when discussing commentary, whether that of Chazal or later scholars. Although the commentators are no longer physically alive, their words are eternally present.

Chazal often use the words of the Torah to uncover a concept which they express in a cryptic, pithy, and obscure way. Many of their statements were frustratingly difficult to understand without further interpretation. Why did they choose to be indirect? If you have something to say, why not just say it?

An essential feature of this Oral Law is its method. It is more than an explanation of the written Torah. It is more than information. It is actually the method of Torah—the process of uncovering truth using your mind. Based on my own observations as a teacher, I understand the method as a way to lead the learner to independently reason through the information.

For example, today I was tutoring algebra. My student and I looked at a problem together before he tackled it. He started solving it in a longer, more cumbersome way than the approach I would have recommended.

I didn't show him how I would have tackled the problem because that would have left a gap in his understanding. If he had had no idea where to begin, I would have taught him my way. But he did have an idea, and his approach eventually led him to the correct answer, albeit by the scenic route. Instead of redirecting him, I looked over his shoulder, and kept him on his chosen track by pointing out when he subtracted instead of dividing.

In a few months, when he sees a similar problem, he will know by himself how to do it the shorter way. This is because he himself will be ready to see it. Before he is ready, I would only confuse him by taking him via the direct route, or give him a mechanical way to solve the problem without understanding why it works, because the solution would not naturally flow out of his own understanding of the material.

Do you see how this example applies to Chazal's commentary on the Torah? Being fed information is not as useful as making the breakthroughs with your own mind. It doesn't feel the same when you finally get it, it doesn't stay in your head the same way, and it isn't *yours*.

Remember what we said about Man's unique nature? The sages designed their statements so that not only would the words contain a concept, but they would also contain the process of acquiring the concept, a process that is naturally enjoyable to human beings because we were designed to perform this type of inquiry.

But wait, there's more. Since Chazal's statements are so cryptic, they contain many potential layers of meaning. When you revisit the same statement, you can always gain more insight.

Conversely, a cryptic statement is like a door with a lock. The insight it imparts is not accessible to people who aren't ready. Gaining insight is a delicate, personal process. Each concept builds on what we already know, and becomes part of our worldview. Hopefully the more we live, the more sophisticated our perspective becomes.

The Theory behind the Jewish Approach to Pain

"It takes a while to get pregnant," you read. "It takes an average of a year." You, of course, can rattle off the names of five women you know who conceived the first month they tried. In fact, I'll bet you know lots of people who conceived while using birth control. I even heard of one woman who conceived each of her children using a different method of birth control.

As the months pass, you begin to wonder if there is a problem. After six months, you consult the doctor. Soon you are reading up on causes and treatments. You are taking hormones and diagnostic tests and snapping at your husband.

There are many excellent resources for researching infertility in a medical framework. You can learn about your uterus, ovaries, fallopian tubes and your LH levels. You can learn about normal and abnormal sperm count and morphology. But where can you go for a systematic approach to coping with the emotional pain of infertility?

Infertility is more than what is happening (or not happening) in your reproductive system. Infertility is a deeply painful situation that can cause you to question the value of your life and the purpose of your existence. But when you are drowning in this quagmire of pain, infertility, if looked at methodically, can be a powerful tool for growth.

An astonishing fact is that all four Matriarchs in the Bible dealt with infertility, and three out of the four coped with primary infertility. This is a comforting thought: God clearly isn't just out to get *you*, since He also afflicted His favored ones with this painful situation. So you have to wonder: is there a point to infertility?

Kick your shoes off and get comfortable. We are about to embark on a journey to answer that question.

Infertility has to be dealt with in a larger context. Infertility is just one of the many types of pain that human beings encounter. If we are interested in how the Torah tells us to handle infertility, it is useful to first address the Torah's approach to pain in general.

Rabbi Joseph B. Soloveitchik (lovingly called *the Rav* by the Orthodox Jewish community), in his book *Fate and Destiny*, suggests a construct that is startlingly useful in its clarity and innovation.[4] I found his questions refreshing for their honesty and his answers practical.

He says that human beings struggle with the problem of suffering in the world. We wonder why. Why did God create the world with so much suffering? How does this fit in with the premise that God is good? If He is good, how can He let this go on? And, on a more personal note, how come, if I'm a more righteous person than the lady down the block, I can't conceive and she has four healthy children?

You may be one of those people who doesn't believe that God intervenes in the lives of individual human beings,[5] in which case you are content to accept the purely physical cause of your infertility as explanation enough. (My personal medical diagnosis was "unexplained infertility," which might well mean that my case had a scientific cause that doctors were unaware of at the time.) That approach might allow you to detour around most of the troubling theological issues. But if you keep reading, I think you may see that this approach still has something to offer you.

The classic approach to our philosophical conundrum is to try to explain that evil and suffering are not truly evil.

"This must be happening for a reason." (What reason? You spend hours thinking about it.)

"I must somehow deserve this." (Why? What did you do? You think about it for hours.)

"All of this will work out for the best." (You construct a scenario where, without your having suffered, for example, having been injured in a car accident and undergone reconstructive surgery and rehabilitative therapy, you wouldn't have met the man you ultimately married and lived happily-ever-after with.)

Although these approaches work for some people, I'm not going to go into the difficulties each one presents. Instead, let's turn to the elegant simplicity of the Rav.

The Rav takes a different path. "Judaism, with its realistic approach to man and his place in the world, understood that evil cannot be blurred or camouflaged."[6] I like that. Rav Soloveitchik does not deny evil. He does not avoid calling a spade a spade. "Evil is an undeniable fact. There is evil, there is suffering, there are hellish torments in this world." Yes, there are! Thank you for having the guts to say so!

How is the Rav able to do this and still maintain that God is good? He performs a neat little move with huge ramifications.

The Rav makes a distinction between the world from the perspective of the Almighty Creator and the perspective of the human creation. To us, the creations, there is awful and painful evil. Any attempt to downplay this will fail. Whoever tries to delude himself by romanticizing human existence is nothing but a fool. It is impossible to overcome the hideousness of evil by trying to understand it.[7] Any attempt to try to overcome the hideousness of evil through understanding it will fail! *Fail*!

The Rav then explains that from the perspective of the Creator, there is no evil. "Certainly, the testimony of the Torah that the cosmos is very good is true. However, this affirmation may be made only from the infinite perspective of the Creator. Finite man, with his partial vision, cannot uncover the absolute good in the cosmos..."[8]

Got that? From God's perspective, it's not evil. While it may be comforting for us to believe that God knows what He is doing, it can still leave us in a mental bind—we may never be able to understand this apparent contradiction. But Man is absolved from doing all sorts of mental gymnastics to try to comprehend it. We will fail.

You may think that means that Man is stuck. Any time we posit that Man can't understand something, it could be an easy cop-out for Man to say, "Oh, sorry, I can't be held responsible; my feeble brain can't comprehend that."

Not so fast.

The beauty of the Rav's approach is that he takes us out of unproductive self-flagellation and moves us towards a truly practical solution.

As we said, mankind is caught in a bind. "Only if Man could grasp the world as a whole would he be able to gain a perspective on the essential nature of evil." However, since it is impossible for Man to grasp the world as a whole, "...Judaism determined that Man...will seek in vain for the solution to the problem of evil within the framework of speculative thought, for he will never find it."[9]

So what is Man to do? God may be just, but Man experiences it as evil. The Rav offers us the solution. He calls it the *halachic* approach. *Halacha* comes from the Hebrew root "to walk" or "to move forward."[10]

"Evil exists, and I will neither deny it nor camouflage it with vain intellectual gymnastics. I am concerned about evil from a halachic standpoint, like a person who wishes to know the deed which he shall do; I ask one simple question: what must the sufferer do so that he may live through his suffering?"[11]

Instead of emphasizing the *why*, Judaism emphasizes the *what*. Instead of agonizing over why this is happening, the Rav suggests that a person reflect on what to do. "The fundamental question is: what obligation does suffering impose upon man?"[12]

Reflect carefully and appreciate the freedom that this answer gives you. In this way, Man frees himself from asking a question that has no answer. He can cease to struggle with the tormenting question of how God can allow this to happen.

And yet, his responsibilities have just begun. Because, although only God can know the *why*, there is still a large realm accessible to Man. And that is the realm of Man himself. Instead of focusing on Man's feeble perceptions of God's responsibilities to him, he can turn his focus inward.

As Rav Soloveitchik writes, "We do not inquire about the hidden ways of the Almighty, but, rather, about the path wherein man shall walk when suffering strikes. We ask about neither the cause of evil nor its purpose, but rather how it might be mended and elevated. How shall a person act in a time of trouble? What ought a man to do so that he not perish in his affliction?

"The halachic answer to this question is very simple. Afflictions come to elevate a person, to purify and sanctify his spirit, to cleanse and purge it of the dross of superficiality and vulgarity, to refine his soul and to broaden his horizons. In a word, the function of suffering is to *mend* that which is flawed in an individual's personality."[13]

According to the Rav's explanation, pain does not necessarily occur because God is directly punishing a person for specific sins. Rather, pain can change a person. A person can reflect on the pain he feels and ferret out the distortions and misconceptions that he holds. The pain in any situation can help a person discover and reflect on the flaws in his character. The difficulties he encounters can cause him to isolate these defects and refine his character, which he may never before have needed to confront in a previously comfortable, cushy existence.

Let us now examine infertility in this framework.

Applying This Theory to Infertility

So now we have an approach. Infertility causes pain. We are not going discuss *why* it is happening. (Scientifically, either you know why or you don't. Theologically, unless a prophet tells you why, you will never know.)[14] We will proceed on the premise that pain *can* lead to emotional growth.

But pain does not always lead to growth. People can be crushed by pain, contradicting another myth that minimizes the evilness of evil: "God only gives us what we can handle." What do we say about those who don't handle it? How do we explain all the people driven to mental illness by the great pain in their lives that they cannot manage?

Human beings are complex creatures. Why do some people seem to grow stronger from coping with suffering, and some grow weaker?

("He never was the same after his six-year-old son was run over by that car.") Some people gain insight and new perspective. Some grow bitter.

I'm not going to try to isolate the factors. I will say this: right now you are in pain.

You have a tool. You have a brain capable of abstract thought and reflection. You have feelings. And you can think about those feelings. Using your mind to think about your feelings is the key to growth.

What do I mean?

If you walk into a room and someone hands you an apron, a cap, a bucket full of Spackle, three smooth stones, a rope, and a brush, what will you do with it? Your answer will depend on the purpose you want to achieve. If your goal is home improvement, you will use those objects differently than if your goal is to put on a play to amuse a cancer patient.

So you have a purpose. Your purpose is to use your pain to grow.

Now all you need is education. If your purpose is home improvement, you need a lesson on the uses of Spackle and brushes in redecorating. If your purpose is entertainment, you need education on the comedic uses of rope.

Your purpose is growth. You need education on the uses of pain for self-improvement.

The amazing crescendo in this logical build-up is that the Bible can provide an education on the uses of infertility for growth.

All you need is the following guide, your feelings, and your mind.

---

[1] Not to be confused with middle-aged.

[2] Maimonides' third reason to believe a source was if it was attested to by "tradition derived from the prophets and the righteous." The Jews haven't had a prophet for almost two thousand years. There are strict, explicit, undeniable criteria that must be fulfilled in order for a person to qualify as a prophet: you must exactly predict an event, or perform a supernatural act, as proof that God has spoken to you. (Deuteronomy 13:2 and 18:21-22)

3 Paraphrase of Maimonides *Letter on Astrology/Letter to the Jews of Marseilles*.

4 His approach was new to me; the Rav offers an approach that I had never encountered before during my "mainstream" Jewish education.

5 Many great Jewish thinkers maintain that the majority of people are generally subject to the laws of nature, not under the specific intervention of God.

6 Rabbi Joseph B. Soloveitchik, *Fate and Destiny*, page 4.

7 Ibid. This is a paraphrase; the original uses words like "naught," "fantast," and "philosophico-speculative."

8 Ibid, pp. 4-5.

9 Ibid, p. 5.

10 *Halacha* is the Hebrew word Jews use for the Laws God gave. When we ask of our rabbi, "What is the *halacha*?" it literally means "What is the way to go?" but is used in the sense of "What is the law in this situation?"

11 Soloveitchik, p. 7.

12 Ibid., p. 7.

13 Ibid, p. 8

14 One of the clearest demonstrations of this concept from the Bible is in the Book of Esther. Esther, a Jewish girl, is chosen over all of the girls in the kingdom to be the queen. She just happens to be the cousin and adopted daughter of Mordechai, a Jewish leader. When, a few years later, a decree goes forth that all Jews in the kingdom will be obliterated—amazingly, the Jews have an advocate, the queen, right in the palace! Doesn't this seem like too many coincidences to say it just happened by chance? Isn't it tempting to claim, "God clearly planned all of this for a purpose?" Mordechai comes to tell Esther to go before the king and beg for mercy on behalf of the Jewish people. Esther is hesitant to go see the king without an appointment, as her adoptive father suggests. Mordechai answers her (Esther 4:14): "Who knows whether it was for a situation like this that you attained the royal position?" *Who knows*? Even with all those coincidences, Mordechai says we must still speculate as to their purpose. (And of course, act appropriately as reason dictates.)

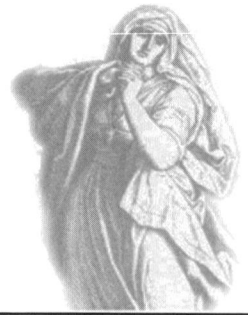

Chapter II

How the Matriarchs Coped with Infertility

The content of the Torah can be divided into two main categories: laws and stories.

Laws are concepts formulated as actions that can have an effect on a person. There is one major law relating to infertility, and that is: "And God said to them: 'Be fruitful and multiply.'" (Genesis 1:28.)

This is not exactly a law.[1] It is a general indication of God's will at the time He was speaking to Adam and Eve. As God seems to indicate that He is in favor of procreation, we will address this issue later, after we've devoted some chapters to the stories of the Matriarchs.

Now for stories. As I mentioned before, three of the four Matriarchs—Sarah, Rebecca, and Rachel—experienced infertility, and even the fourth, the most fertile Matriarch, Leah, experienced a stretch of time when she had some difficulty conceiving.

> "And Sarai was barren; she had no child." (Genesis 11:30.)
>
> "And Isaac prayed to God opposite his wife [Rebecca] because she was barren." (Genesis 25:21.)
>
> "And God saw that Leah was hated, and He opened her womb, and Rachel was barren." (Genesis 29:31.)

I have some questions to pose before we discuss how these three women coped with their infertility:

Was there a purpose to the infertility of the Matriarchs?

If so, *what* was the purpose of their infertility?

If there was a purpose to their infertility, why wasn't Leah, one of the Matriarchs, initially afflicted with infertility?

Assuming there was a particular purpose to the infertility of the Matriarchs, might that same purpose apply to me if my infertility is not providentially determined, but rather a result of the laws of nature?

Leah Is Spared

Methodologically speaking, it would make sense if we could establish that Leah, too, was "supposed" to be infertile, and that it was only because of some other factor (which we would have to explain) that she did not experience primary infertility. Then we could explore the Matriarchs as a category of women subject to infertility.

So we're going to skip ahead a little and look at Leah's story out of order.

How much do you know about Rachel and Leah? Avid Bible readers probably know the story.

The setting: Jacob, Patriarch #3, came to his maternal uncle Lavan's house to escape his twin brother's murderous wrath (fascinating, right?) and to find a wife.

Genesis 29:15-35

> Lavan says to Jacob, "Just because you're my relative, does that mean you should work for free? Tell me your wages." And Lavan had two daughters; the older one's name was Leah, and the younger one's name was Rachel. Leah's eyes were tender (*not sure what that means*) and Rachel was beautiful of form and beautiful of appearance. Jacob loved Rachel, and

he said, "I'll work for you for seven years for Rachel, your younger daughter." Lavan said, "It's better for me to give her to you than to give her to another man; stay with me." (*Was this a backhanded compliment?*)

Jacob worked to earn Rachel for seven years, and in his eyes they were like a few days, because of his love for her. Jacob said to Lavan, "Bring me my wife, because I finished my term, and I will consort with her." And Lavan gathered all the people of the place, and he made a party. And that night, he took Leah his daughter and brought her to him, and he consorted with her. (*Switcheroo!*) And Lavan gave his maidservant Zilpah to Leah, his daughter, as a maidservant. (*Why mention that here?*) And in the morning, behold it was Leah!

And Jacob said to Lavan, "What did you do to me? Didn't I work for you for Rachel? Why did you cheat me?" And Lavan said, "Look, we don't do that in our community—give the younger before the older. Let's finish up this week of partying, and I'll give Rachel to you also, for work you'll do for me for another seven years." And Jacob did that, and finished out the week, and Lavan gave him his daughter Rachel for a wife. (And Lavan gave his maidservant Bilhah to his daughter Rachel as a maidservant.) And Jacob also consorted with Rachel and he also loved Rachel more than Leah; and he worked for Lavan for another seven years.

God saw that Leah was hated and he opened her womb, and Rachel was barren. Leah became pregnant and had a boy, and she called him Reuven [literally, *See, a son!*] because, as Leah said, "God has seen my affliction, and now my husband will love me." She got pregnant again and had a[nother] son and she said, "Because God has heard that I am hated and gave me also him," and she called him Shimon [from the Hebrew root *to hear*]. She became pregnant again and had a [third] son and she said, "Now my husband will be attached to me because I bore him three sons," and she called him Levi [from the root *attach*]. And she became pregnant again and had a [fourth] son and she said, "This time I will gratefully praise God." Therefore she named him Yehuda [*praise/thank God*]. And she stopped giving birth.

Bear in mind that certain subtleties, complexities, and ambiguities are literally lost in translation because you are not reading the text in the original language. But we'll do our best.

The upshot was that Leah found herself in the unhappy position (one which is hard to relate to in our society of one-wife-per-husband, at least at any given time) of being the wife that her husband did not love.

What fascinates me is that a closer reading of the text does not quite bear out that claim. In fact, the text seems to be downright contradictory. I know, it's shocking. Contradictory verses in the Bible?

Verse 31 says, "And God saw that Leah was hated, and He opened her womb, and Rachel was barren." So God Himself saw that Leah was hated. God wouldn't see something that isn't there, would He?

But the Ramban (also known as Nachmanides), a thirteenth century scholar, makes an interesting point. He says that Jacob did not hate Leah. He cites verse 30 to prove it: "And he loved Rachel *more than* Leah." Okay. He loved Rachel *more*. But you can't say Jacob *hated* Leah. He loved her.

So did Jacob hate her? It seems not. Then what exactly was God seeing that caused Him to open her womb?

Before we try to resolve the contradiction, I want to stay with that verse for a moment: "And God saw that Leah was hated, and He opened her womb, and Rachel was barren." What is Rachel doing in this verse? What does she have to do with Leah and God opening Leah's womb? What does it mean that *God* opened her womb? Does God open each woman's womb every time she conceives? Or is an open womb a term for "fertile" and a closed womb for "infertile"?

Sforno, a sixteenth-century Italian commentator, remarks on this. On the words *and Rachel was barren*: "She was barren by nature, and remained that way until the Powerful Blessed One opened her womb," implying that a closed womb is a physically infertile womb. The Torah says that God opened Leah's womb, implying she was barren prior to God's act of "opening" her womb.

Back to our contradiction. Why did God open Leah's womb? It seems that Leah would not have conceived as immediately as she did were it not for God seeing that she was hated. Except that according to verse 30, she was not hated.

Sink your teeth into that one.

It would have been legitimate for Jacob to divorce Leah. He married her under false pretenses. Ramban explains that "God saw," that God had compassion for Leah so that Jacob wouldn't leave her [and therefore opened her womb]. He says that when one wife is greatly beloved, the other is referred to as "hated" in comparison. This was humiliating to Leah and God saw her affliction. Not that Leah was *actually* hated by Jacob, but that it was Leah's *perception*, in comparison with Jacob's feelings for Rachel, that she was hated. This resolves the contradiction. The Torah first records the fact that Jacob loved both Leah and Rachel. Then it records the fact of Leah's feelings—that she felt hated.

So now we have an indication that Leah was subject to the infertility of the Matriarchs, but her infertility was removed because God had compassion for her situation. So you have to wonder: why did God want the Matriarchs to be infertile?

While we're on this subject, let's ask a question to come back to later: if Leah was slated to be infertile, but the plan was changed—how might this apply to us? Is there something we can do to change our own situations? Or is our only option to become "unfavored" wives? And would that even work?

Now that these questions are bugging you (I hope), I'm going to leave them aside for a while. I put the chapters in this order for a reason—I have a systematic build-up here. But I promise we'll get back to it later.

Techniques of the Matriarchs

Caution: this section is mildly technical. I recommend you read it when your brain is functioning optimally.

So far we have established a category of infertile Matriarchs. Before we head into the specific challenges of each individual Matriarch, I'd like to discuss some general points.

The efforts of the Matriarchs in response to their infertility can be divided into two categories: those designed to work through the laws of nature, and those designed to get God to intervene in the laws of nature.

Today's increased medical knowledge and technology give us many more options than the Matriarchs had in regard to working through the laws of nature. We have deeper knowledge of the reproductive system and its hormonal and physical factors. We have the technology to manipulate those factors, which increases the probability of conceiving.

Certainly it makes sense to do everything we can to manipulate the laws of nature in our favor. God told Man: "Fill the earth and conquer it" (Genesis 1:28), which is a reference to mastery over nature through technology. So go to a specialist!!

In those days, medicine was unable to alleviate infertility. Doctors had no options to offer. A woman who was not ovulating had no way to make herself ovulate. A woman with blockages had no way to open them. Sperm that had difficulty reaching its destination had no way to improve its odds.

Although the range of medical options available to the Matriarchs was more limited, it is important to note that they *did* seek medical options. Our Matriarchs made use of the limited medical strategies of their time, as we'll see when we study Rachel.

The second category of endeavor is to try to get God to intervene in the laws of nature. At first, that may sound strange to you. Get God to intervene? Isn't it His choice whether or not He intervenes? And if you don't believe in God at all, or believe in a Creator, but not one that intervenes, it certainly doesn't make sense.

It is one of the fundamental principles of Judaism, as we stated among our premises, that the Creator interacts with His creations. There is actually a method to get God to interact with His creations, in a general way. There are many factors that determine how God runs His universe and we can't get into His head. *"My thoughts* [God's] *are not your thoughts* [Man's]*."* (Isaiah 55:8.)

If, at this point, you are rolling your eyes because of the whole "God intervening" thing, don't close the book just yet. Should you staunchly maintain that God will never, ever intervene no matter what you do, either because He doesn't exist or because He doesn't intervene—which may be a logical position based on strict observation of your life—the Matriarchs still have something to offer. Recall the Rav's words: pain can function to remove the dross of superficiality and vulgarity, to broaden your horizons, to mend that which is flawed in an individual's personality. Even if you don't buy into God, do you admit to the possibility of a few character flaws?

Before we get into the methodology of activating divine intervention, let's discuss a *misconception* on the subject. Skeptics, you should enjoy reading about what is *not* true. This is something on which we will probably agree.

I Do for God and He Does for Me

In this schema, God and I are involved in a symbiosis, a mutually agreeable trade. He gave us the Bible, which has lots of laws and suggestions in it. He wants us or needs us to live by and perform those laws. If we do, He is happy and rewards us by giving us things that we want.

Let's take a look at the underlying assumptions of that schema:

God gave us a set of arbitrary activities to do;

God needs our activities in order for Him to be happy;

God commands painful activities, but if we perform them, He might give us what we really want;

The true good in this life is what *we* really want, not the commandments.

Here is an alternate approach:

God gave us a set of activities that are designed to increase our understanding of ourselves and the world around us;

God lacks nothing, and we cannot "get" Him by violating or ignoring His commandments. The only thing that happens is that we lose the opportunity to gain insight into ourselves and the world. Or we become further entrenched in a distorted view of the world around us;

The best thing we can achieve in this life is an understanding of the principles behind it. There is no reward for that. Understanding is its own reward because it leads to the benefit of a successful life;

Any "reward" can only be deeper understanding or the opportunity for deeper insight.

I imagine that everyone agrees that understanding how life works is the key to navigating through it with success. So even if you spend your whole life trying to gain understanding, and God never once responds to you and intervenes on your behalf, you'll *still* be in a better position for success with knowledge than without knowledge.

The method for demonstrating which schema is correct is quite simple. The first schema may seem correct from a superficial look at the commandments. But try studying the commandments with the premise that every single one is designed to increase our understanding of ourselves and the world around us.[2] Each insight that you gain is a demonstration.

That being said, we can begin to discuss divine intervention.

Does divine intervention work according to a methodical system? Or does God decide on a case-by-case basis?

What *can* we know about it? Or what can we rule out? Often, ruling out possibilities makes things much clearer.

A word to any agnostics—it's logical to think that God would not break the laws of nature. When God told Abraham that He would bless him and his wife with a son, in Genesis 17:17, "Abraham fell on his face and laughed in joy; and he thought, 'A child born to a centenarian?! And will Sarah—a ninety-year-old—give birth?!?'" Abraham may have been happy, but he certainly was surprised.

Divine intervention is not determined by reason alone. We know this because God communicated to us that He intervenes. Without Him telling us that, we wouldn't necessarily be able to deduce it logically.[3]

In the Torah, there are lots of descriptions of God: merciful, vengeful, jealous, generous, et al. Many of these attributes are contradictory.

This doesn't bother us that much because humans are plenty contradictory. And assuming God is just a super-human, why shouldn't He be moody and emotional like the rest of us?

Maintaining this position gets a little tricky when we try to square it with the Jewish premise of God's Oneness. "Hear O Israel, the Lord is our God, the Lord is ONE" (Deuteronomy 6:4.)

Judaism maintains that God's ONEness is unique. He is not subject to parts—that would be more than one. Primarily, this means He is not physical, because then He would be divisible into parts.[4]

A vital corollary of this is that God does not have emotions.[5] He doesn't *have* anything. Because then there would be Him and his emotions. Two separate things—parts again. If He's happy, then sad, or loving, then angry, then He's changing. Changing means first one thing, then another. Not One.

This may seem somewhat confusing. It helps if you don't try to grasp what God *is*, if He's One. Focus on ruling out. *God looks like an old man with a white beard,* you muse to yourself. *No, wait a minute. That contradicts the concept of One. God can't have a beard. That would be parts—Him and a beard.* And so on.

If God has no parts, how am I supposed to follow a method that gets Him to change His mind? First, He decides I'm infertile. Then, He decides I shouldn't be infertile. Changing is first one thing, then another. Parts!

Jewish premise: we cannot change God. God does not change. Yet, somehow, we can effectuate divine intervention. How?

A wonderful metaphor that explains this is fire.[6] The fire stays the same. Different metals that you place in front of the fire react differently. One metal turns green. Another metal sparks. One compound melts. Another one hardens. *The fire remains the same.* How the object is affected by the fire depends on the nature of the object. Change its nature, and the effects of its interaction with the fire will change, without the fire changing at all. That works for Man's relationship with God, too. God doesn't change. When you are an X-type person, God relates to you in an X-type way. And X events occur. If you become a Y-type person, then Y events occur, without God changing at all.

Here's another illustration. You look around. All you see are shadowy dark, blurry, shapes. Then you get eye surgery. You can see colors. You put on glasses—suddenly you see sharp, crisp, images. You put on infrared glasses. You can "see" heat! Look at the world through a microscope, and you can see cells. Look through a really powerful microscope, and you can see atoms! The amazing thing is that the world doesn't have to do anything. It can just sit there, twiddling its anthropomorphic thumbs, and it can change drastically while *not changing at all*!

Change yourself, and around you, the world will change.

---

[1] Although, according to Oral Law, this is the basis of the technical obligation for every Jewish male to father a minimum of one boy child and one girl child. But the exegesis that determines the orally passed down laws does not negate the plain meaning of the text.

[2] A good teacher is helpful in unlocking this wisdom.

[3] I claim that it *is* logical to maintain that what is written in the Bible is true. You can write to me if you want to discuss this point—it's too big a topic to cover in a footnote.

[4] Maimonides, Laws of the Fundamentals of the Torah 1:7.

[5] Maimonides, Laws of the Fundamentals of the Torah 1:11. If you're wondering about all the stuff in the Bible like God getting angry and rejoicing and being sad, Maimonides explains it in Law 12.

[6] This metaphor comes from Maimonides' *Guide to the Perplexed* (Moreh Nevuchim).

Chapter III

Sarah

Let's do a little math.

When we first meet Abraham and Sarah (still known by their earlier names Abram and Sarai, before God changed their names in Genesis 17:5 and 17:15), God tells Abraham to leave his current land and go to Canaan (currently Israel). Abram was age seventy-five at the time. (Genesis 12:4.)

God tells Abram that He is going to make his descendents into a great nation. (See Genesis 12:2, 12:7, 13:15-16, 15:4, 15:18.) God and Abram make a covenant that Abram's offspring will inherit the land of Canaan.

We don't know how long Abram and Sarai were married before we met them. According to the Bible, Abram had his first son, Ishmael, when he was eighty-six. (Genesis 16:16.) Abraham and Sarah had a son together, Isaac, when he was a hundred and she was ninety. (Genesis 17:1, 17:17, and 18:10—look it up and do the math if you think I miscalculated.)

We met them when Abram was seventy-five. Abraham and Sarah had a child together when he was a hundred and she was ninety. That gave them a minimum of twenty-five years of barrenness, assuming they were newlyweds when we met them, at ages seventy-five and sixty-five, which I, personally, find unlikely.

Exploring the Option of "Child-free" Living

Sarah's situation seems different from those of the other Matriarchs. Rachel and Rebecca try to have children, as we'll discuss in their chapters. But Sarah treats her infertility differently. The text reports no steps taken by Sarah in an attempt to bear children until God tells Abraham that he will have children.[1] Abraham asks (Genesis 15:2-6):

> "What can you give me when I am childless and the steward of my household is Eliezer the Damascene?" And Abram said, "See, you haven't given me offspring, and behold my steward is my heir." [Repetitive?] And behold, the word of God came to him, saying, "He will not inherit you; rather, what will come forth from within you will inherit you." And He took him outside and said, "Please look at the sky and count the stars if you can count them." And He said to him, "Like this will be your offspring." And he believed in God, and He considered it for him righteousness.

God makes a covenant with Abraham promising him children. It was this covenant that triggered Sarah's first recorded effort to have children.

I want to point out that God intervened in the laws of nature as they affected Abram's and Sarai's lives because He was establishing a nation, using Abram as the Patriarch and Sarai as the Matriarch. They had the qualities that He wanted to use as role models for His nation. Had God not intervened, apparently Abraham and Sarah would have lived out their lives childless: "And Abraham and Sarah were old, well on in years; the flow of women had ceased to be for Sarah." (Genesis 18:11.) It was not until Abraham was told explicitly that the nation would come from his genes that Sarah began her efforts to ensure that he would have offspring. God's intervention in the laws of nature appears to be mission-related, not personal—the rest of us are not in that situation. It is unlikely that this option would be open to us.

So what were Abraham and Sarah doing, if they weren't having children? They seem to have been coping, living their lives without children. When Abram leaves Haran to go to Canaan, he takes his wife, his nephew, and "the souls they had made in Haran." (Genesis 12:5.) Rashi, an eleventh-century commentator, discusses the strange term "made." How do you make a person? Or make a soul? Isn't that God's job?

Rashi says that Sarai spoke to the women and Abram to the men. By opening their eyes to the nature of the universe and how Man's nature interacts with it, in a sense they gave these people life. Genesis 21:33 gives us a little hint as to their approach:

"He planted an *eshel* in Beer Sheva, and there he proclaimed the name of God, Master of the Universe." The Rabbis in the Talmud interpret *eshel* in two ways;[2] either it was an orchard planted in the desert to provide relief for travelers, or it was an inn (*E'Sh'L* being an acronym for three Hebrew words which mean "eating, drinking, and sleeping"). Abraham cared deeply about all of humanity and set up an oasis in the desert for weary travelers. There he would engage people in philosophical discussions about whether or not there was a Creator. We will discuss this further, later.

So until about age eighty-five, Abraham and Sarah were living "child-free."

My use of quotes around the term "child-free" tells you that I am using it tongue-in-cheek. If you're reading this, you probably don't view your situation as giving you a certain freedom. More likely, it chains you, weighing obsessively on your mind.

I remember reading the material my doctor gave me in preparation for the IUI (intra-uterine-insemination) procedure. It discussed my doses of medication, how, where, and when to apply them, the daily appointments, blood tests, and sonograms. I knew I was up to my second-to-last medical option (the final option being IVF, in-vitro fertilization).

One of the pages in the folder listed further options in the event that IUI failed. "Try IUI again. Make the move to IVF. Adoption." The final bullet on the page read, "Explore the option of child-free living."

That smug, bulleted option sent me over the edge. Child-free?! Child-FREE?! I swiped my face with my sleeve and snarled at the word "Explore" as the print on the page was blurred by a teardrop.

I wasn't child-FREE, I was child-LESS, and I didn't want to be child-FREE, I wanted to be child-FULL. I resented their trying to reframe my situation in a more positive way. I didn't want to think positively about my infertility, to grow resigned to the emptiness, and to look at the bright side.

And I felt it was the height of insensitivity to imply that I, a woman who was about to puncture herself daily for eleven days after practicing on an orange, should really get past this little "issue" about not having children, and go off and enjoy my freedom.

Now, years later, I think I see what they were getting at. I don't take back my initial reaction. I was a normal hormonal, over-reactive, infertile woman who didn't want to see "child-free" literature in her IUI folder.

But I see now what infertility can do to a person. I see the obsession, from my own experience of infertility. Human beings have a tremendous amount of energy. When you direct all of your energy into one area, you have prodigious resources at your disposal. But right now, all that energy is tied up in wanting pregnancy. If you don't reframe your situation positively, you can end up being a slave to your infertility, and all that powerful energy will go to waste.

Life is more than having a child or children. I know you don't believe me. What I mean is that you know that life is more than having a child, but at the same time you don't believe me, because you are spending all your energy in this one area. And maybe you won't have to believe me. Maybe your treatments will work and you'll have your baby/ies and move on from the time in your life when all you thought about was getting pregnant.

But if you can look at this time as a gift, a valuable period in your life when you have few if any burdens and obligations to children—you will have time and you will have energy. If you do end up being child-free ultimately, you will be in a situation where you can choose how you want to focus your life. What would you like to do with the time and energy that is yours to invest? You don't have to waste your precious resources reading and thinking and crying about infertility! (I mean after you finish reading this book, of course.)

Easy for her to say, you're thinking. I understand that an infertile woman's energy naturally flows towards the subject of her infertility. But to the extent that I am able to pull myself out of my preoccupation with infertility and concentrate on my freedom and what I want to do with it, my infertile years are serving me well.

Sarah's Choice

Once God had made a covenant with Abraham that the nation would be based on his biological child, Sarah took action. As we've discussed, Sarah (or any other woman of that time period) didn't have many medical options open to her.

Genesis 16:1-4 says:
> And Sarai the wife of Abram had borne him no children; and she had an Egyptian maidservant and her name was Hagar. Sarai said to Abram, "Behold, God has stopped me from giving birth; consort please with my maidservant—maybe I will be built up from her." And Abram listened to Sarai's voice. And Sarai the wife of Abram took Hagar the Egyptian, her maidservant (after Abram had been living in the land of Canaan for ten years), and gave her to Abram her husband, as a wife. He consorted with Hagar and she got pregnant. And

when she saw that she had become pregnant, her mistress became light (degraded) in her eyes.

Well, that's a mouthful, as usual. Before we go on, take a moment to formulate some questions (you can't really approach any verse in the Bible without asking questions, though I certainly don't promise to answer them). You might want to fold down the corner of this page (unless it's from the library) because we'll be coming back to these verses over the next few chapters.

All right, do you have your questions? Here are some of mine:

What's this thing about giving Abram another wife?

What does it mean, "Maybe I'll be built up from her?"

What's the "wife of Abram" and "Abram, her husband" stuff? We know who they are already; we've known them for ten years.

Why did Hagar look down on Sarai?

And a general question:

Is this Sarai's plan to have children? God told Abram he would have children in the covenant. Did Sarai deduce that it meant him, not her? Why didn't Abram take another wife? Why was the action initiated by Sarai? (Were any of these your questions? Did I miss any?)

Before we dive into the whole Sarah/Hagar thing, I want to address an important point that the Torah mentions tangentially while discussing Sarah.

The Pain of Infertility

I want to highlight a poignant Rashi commentary. Rashi, who comments on almost every single verse in the Torah, includes select quotes from *Chazal* in addition to elucidating the plain meaning of the text.

Let's take a look back at verse 16:2. "Sarai said to Abram, 'Behold, God has stopped me from giving birth; please consort with my maidservant, maybe I will be built up from her.' And Abram listened to the voice of Sarai his wife."

On the words "maybe I will be built up from her," Chazal comment: "We learn that whoever has no children is not built, rather broken."

Pithy and cryptic. What do you make of it?

Again, the key to unlocking the meaning is to ask questions which will point us toward finding answers. Hopefully, by the end of the chapter, we will have arrived at some.

Why does having children make you "built"?

Why does a lack of children make you "broken"?

In what way are you broken?

Is this "brokenness" in a physical, spiritual, or psychological sense?

What are Chazal trying to convey with this? Is it just a way of saying, "Infertile people are in pain?" Where is the insight in that?

All right, enough questions for now.

I hesitate to take the psychological approach. While "broken" might refer to the emotional effect of being childless, I think Chazal are describing a brokenness that is more than just emotional. After we flesh out this concept, we may even reach some insight as to what makes the childless state so painful.

Which question should we answer first? Let's go back to our first question. What does "building" have to do with having children?

To answer that, let's take a brief foray into Deuteronomy 25:5-11:

> When brothers live together and one of them dies, and he has no child, the wife of the dead shall not marry outside to a strange man; her brother-in-law shall come to her and take her as a wife and perform levirate marriage. And the firstborn that she gives birth to will uphold the name of his dead brother, and his name will not be erased from Israel. But if the man doesn't want to marry his sister-in-law, then his sister-in-law will go up to the gate to the elders, and she will say, "My brother-in-law refuses to establish a name for his brother in Israel; he does not want to perform levirate marriage with me." And the elders of his city call him and speak to him,

and he will stand and say, "I don't want to marry her." And his sister-in-law will approach him before the eyes of the elders, and she will take his shoe off of his foot and spit before him, and she will answer and say: "This is done to the man who will not *build the house of* his brother." And his name will be called in Israel, "The *house of* the one whose shoe was removed." (Emphases mine.)

As usual, incredibly fascinating and practically incomprehensible. I can't resist asking more questions. What kind of institution is this? What is its purpose? Why does she take off his shoe and spit? Why is he called *the house of the one whose shoe was removed*? And how would you call him that, anyway? "Hey, Joe—I mean, House of the one whose shoe was removed..."

I direct you to the words that I emphasized: *build the house of*. Same terminology as Chazal's commentary! So here is an answer to our first question. *Having children builds one's house.*

One more source, and then we can begin our analysis. In Exodus 1:21, Pharaoh ordered the Hebrew midwives to kill newborn baby boys on the delivery table. The midwives feared God and defied Pharaoh; in fact they worked hard to make sure that the babies would survive. Imagine the strength it must have taken to stand up to the king! Verse 21 describes the result of their awe of God: "And it was because the midwives feared God that He made them houses."

What are these "houses?" Did God magically erect palaces for the midwives to live in? Rashi explains that houses are *dynasties*.[3] The Hebrew midwives in Egypt were the forebears of the kingship and the priesthood.

The kings and priests of Israel needed to have certain leadership qualities. In fact, entitlement to the status of priesthood and kingship descended from Levi and Judah, [not from Reuven, Israel (Jacob's) firstborn,] meaning they were based on merit, not birth order. The midwives possessed important characteristics: the fear of God, the moral clarity to value truth over social pressure, and the courage to act consistently with their principles—all qualities of leadership. Their "houses" followed from their qualities.

So here are the facts we have so far: Having children builds some sort of house. A house is a dynasty. A house has something to do with the qualities of the person who founds it.

Back to the levirate marriage. What is the brother building for his dead brother? He is building his name, his house; in short, his line.

Why is the Torah so concerned when a line ends? A whole institution is set up to preserve the name of the brother whose line would otherwise end! I don't mean to detract from the significance of a line ending; to the individual whose line ends, it's tragic. But I would have been surprised if the Law dealt with it based only from the perspective of personal tragedy. There must be another element besides the personal tragedy and pain. A "line" must have an objective value.

What do I mean by "personal value" as opposed to "objective value?"

How I decorate my home has personal value. The furniture I choose, the colors, the pictures, all contribute to the feeling of the home. This affects only a small group of people—my family, friends, and visitors. The mood of the decor affects the mood of the inhabitants, so it is valuable, but valuable in a small and limited sphere.

What is objectively valuable? Something like medical research. Medical advances save lives.[4] Although the researcher may be doing research because he or she is personally driven to find the answer, and it can be personally satisfying, medical research has an objective value as well. To put it more concisely, something of objective value benefits mankind as a whole. It helps further the purpose of existence.[5]

Let's get back to why a person's line is important to humanity. Step one: people who have children are built. Step two: being built has something to do with the house, name, or line that you build. Step three: if the Torah institutionalizes it, it must have value. Step four:

building a line is valuable.

So what is the value of a line?

The midwives showed us that a line has to do with the values and ideals of a person.

To be human means abstract thought tucked into a physical body. If you're human, you have a body and you can think. We humans seek to understand and live in the world around us. Because all humans have this in common, there is a common way that we all approach life. But the details of what we do depend on our talents, energies, and capabilities—and values.

And that's where the line comes in. All of humanity is made up of people. People come in lots of different flavors, and each person's contribution is significant to the whole rich tapestry of humanity. If your line is broken, your thread in that tapestry is not complete.

So we've shown that having a line is valuable. Just to put the whole thing together, what aspect of a line is building, and what part of not having a line makes a person broken?

Since human beings think abstractly, all of our activities have a transcendent sense to them. We don't just build structures, we build skyscrapers. We don't just have children, we build dynasties. We don't wear clothing, we design fashion. Man seeks the eternal and immortal in every field of achievement.

In that same way, a person's life is not just about the actual, physical years of his life. Part of the significance of the life that a human being builds is that it spans the generations. Your life is more than your physical life span when you pass your unique way of understanding reality on to the next generation. When your life stops with you, it is, in a sense, broken; your line has been broken off.

Well, that's a downer. If we didn't already feel bad enough about our infertility, now we can add that it's an objective loss to humanity.

For Sarah especially, who was involved in a specific mission, we can see plainly that having no descendants would have been a real loss to humanity. She and Abraham lived in a world of idolatry and wanted to introduce the concept of a direct relationship with one Creator. In a world where people's fear and insecurity drove them to create rituals intended to give them some control over their lives, Abraham and Sarah were teaching a different way. "These rituals are only psychologically meaningful," they said, "they may feel like they'll work, but something that is a figment of your imagination can't truly affect what will happen to you."

Imagine Sarah and Abraham's pain. Their mission is going well. People are beginning to see the difference between deities that their own imaginations create, and the actual Creator. But to really get this project off the ground, to establish a legacy that will last beyond their lifetimes...

"And Abram said, 'My Lord, God. What can You give me while I am childless? ...You have given no offspring, and my steward will inherit me.'" (Genesis 15:2-3.)

Let's look into Sarah's quest for a biological child.

Sarah and Hagar

Sarah and the later Matriarchs all understood that it was important for their husbands to have children to carry on the family mission. Wouldn't most founders of a family business prefer for a well-qualified child to take over the reins when they retire, as opposed to a random well-qualified outsider? This holds as true in the modern world as it was in the days of the Bible, and for good reason; "family managers are far more loyal and passionate about their work than any hired hand."[6]

Surrogate Motherhood?

> "Sarai said to Abram, "Behold, God has stopped me from giving birth; consort please with my maidservant—maybe I will be built up from her."

(If you want to review the rest of this passage, it's earlier in the chapter, where I suggested that you fold down the page.)

What exactly is Sarah's plan?

Sarah is giving her husband her maidservant. This maidservant will be Abraham's wife. When Hagar and Abram have a child, Sarah will be "built up" through that child.

Rav Hirsch (late 1800s) sums it up nicely: "In giving you my own maid, I will have the right to bring the child up. And even though I can't claim to be the actual *physical* originator of the child, I will still be the next closest thing to it—the *cause of its existence and the means of its spiritual development*. That way I will fit myself in and become part of the building of the 'house,' and in this child and its children I will live on."

So in a pragmatic and hopeful move, Sarah plans to transform her lifetime work into a legacy that will carry on through the generations. She plans to participate in the raising of another woman's child with her husband.

In contemporary terms, when one partner is able to have children but the other is not, doctors can facilitate the birth of a baby with the genetic material of one of the parents. The choice to have a child with half of the couple's genetic material and half from someone else is not an easy one. Many people might legitimately feel that it would only be *his* or *her* child, not *mine*.[7]

But Sarah did not let this feeling control her actions. For Sarah to be so strongly committed to her life's work that she would participate in any way she could to ensure its success says something about her character. We will soon see exactly how challenging that was. But first, let's observe something about Abraham and Sarah's marriage.

A Husband's Sensitivity

Abraham would not have chosen this route on his own initiative. He did not suggest taking another wife when his wife Sarah could not have a child. Rav Hirsch comments that it is clear that he was against this plan because Sarah entreated him: *"Please consort with my maidservant."* (Verse 2.) Sarah was thinking of Abraham, but since she knew he wouldn't do it for his own sake, she focused on how much it would mean to her: "Maybe *I* will be built up." If Abraham wasn't willing to do it for himself, she hoped he would do it for her sake, because she wanted it badly.

Abraham did not expect Hagar to provide him with the heir to his mission. Rav Hirsch points out that Verse 2 says, "And Abram listened to the voice of Sarai." *Not* to "the voice of his wife." *Not* because she was his wife and wanted to provide him with children (my interpretation) by the technique Sarah had in mind. He agreed because he wanted to satisfy her personal desire. "He did it for her sake, as she did it for his, a relationship we find repeatedly between Abraham and Sarah, and which are universally to be found where man and woman are true husband and wife together."[8]

Let's see how this played out.

The "Other" Woman

The Torah, with sensitive appreciation of something that we cannot even relate to in this society, refers to the second wife as a *tzara*, which literally means "adversary." This demonstrates explicit understanding that a situation involving multiple wives is inherently competitive.

The book *Siblings Without Rivalry* has an exercise that gives us an inkling of how a wife sharing her husband might feel.[9]

> Imagine that your spouse puts an arm around you and says, "Honey, I love you so much, and you're so wonderful that I've decided to have another wife just like you."
>
> Your reaction:
> _____

When the new wife finally arrives, you see that she's very young and kind of cute. When the three of you are out together, people say "hello" to you politely, but exclaim ecstatically over the newcomer. "Isn't she adorable! Hello sweetheart...You are precious!" Then they turn to you and ask, "How do you like the new wife?"

Your reaction:

_____

The new wife is maturing rapidly. Every day she seems smarter and more competent. One afternoon as you're struggling to figure out the directions on the new computer your husband bought you, she bursts into the room and says, "Oooh, can I use it? I know how."

Your reaction:

_____

When you tell her she can't use it, she runs crying to your husband. Moments later she returns with him. Her face is tear-stained and he has his arm around her. He says to you, "What would be the harm in letting her have a turn? Why can't you share?"

Your reaction:

_____

One day you find your husband and the new wife lying on the bed together. He's tickling her and she's giggling. Suddenly the phone rings and he answers it. Afterwards he tells you that something important has come up and he must leave immediately. He asks you to stay home with the new wife and make sure she's all right.

Your reaction:

_____

According to Jewish Law, in societies where having a second wife was common, it was permitted to Jews as well. In our society, where this doesn't happen except among Mormons, taking a second wife is prohibited out of sensitivity to the women. However, even in those times where it *was* permitted, certain laws applied. Two wives cannot live in the same house.[10] The husband must provide separate households. He must be able to adequately provide food, clothing, and sexual satisfaction to his wives. These laws ease some of the practical conflicts of having two wives, but the above exercise paints a picture of the visceral competition that still would be involved.

Sarah's situation is slightly different because she gives Abraham her maidservant (another institution that we can't relate to), which means she is still Hagar's employer.

However, as soon as Hagar conceives, she begins to look down on Sarah, which ultimately leads to a disagreement between Abraham and Sarah. Without going into the nature of the argument, suffice it to say that God steps in and tells Abraham to listen to Sarah his wife.[11]

We have to ask the question: Why did Hagar look down on Sarah? Martin E. Seligman, in *The Optimistic Child*, explains that a feeling is the result of a thought.[12] Hagar's feelings about Sarah were based on her thoughts.

What did Hagar think? When Hagar degrades Sarah, she is basing her conclusion on unsound logic. Her assumption is this: if you are doing the right thing, God will make you successful.

Rashi comments on 16:4, on the words *Her mistress became lower in her eyes*: Hagar said, "Sarah's hidden self is not as she appears. She presents herself as a righteous woman, and she is not a righteous woman. She didn't merit pregnancy all these years, and I got pregnant on the first try."

Hagar made a common assumption. It's the kind of assumption that hurts us when we make it about others, and hurts us when we make it about ourselves.

She assumed that if a person is unsuccessful in an endeavor, then it must be because he or she is a bad person, or a sinner, or not divinely favored—however you want to put it.

Reward and punishment is one of the fundamental principles of Judaism, but Hagar's assumption is based on a simplistic reading of reward and punishment: if I am good, God rewards me; if I am bad, God punishes me. People often turn this around: If good things are happening to me, it must mean I'm a good person. If bad things are happening, it must mean I'm a bad person.

The Torah teaches that it is incorrect to make deductions based on your situation. If things are going well, it is not necessarily correct to deduce that you are a good person and that God is in favor of your activities. Also, if things are going badly, it is not necessarily correct to assume that God is sending you a message that He doesn't like how you've been behaving. Likewise, when you make these assumptions about others, you are judging them, and it's often just an excuse to feel superior to them. When you make these assumptions about yourself, you can easily become overwhelmed with guilt because you can't figure out what you have done wrong, as opposed to your friends who seem to behave similarly to you and yet don't appear to have the same suffering in their lives.

Great. If I can't make deductions from my situation, then how do I know if God does or doesn't approve of what I'm doing? And if it's not true that these things are messages, then how does reward and punishment work?

It is not sound practice to evaluate your actions by the results. Let's say I try to murder someone, but I end up shooting the wall of his house instead, and a hidden cache of jewels falls out, making him rich for life. Am I justified in concluding that my act of intended murder was good? It may have had positive results, but it doesn't change the fact that I am an aggressive, out-of-control person who feels that it's okay to take someone's life. We would all love to be told whether or not we're being good or bad, as if there was some cosmic scorecard we could look up on the Internet at www.heavenhell.com. But the fact is that it's not that simple. We evaluate the situation and do the best we can. If you want to know whether what you did was right or wrong, ask someone insightful and objective.

Fine. But where does reward and punishment come into this? Aren't good things in my life rewards for being good? And bad things punishments for being bad?

No. And also yes.

Reward and punishment are not a substitute for the laws of nature. Statistically, people with higher education do better financially than people who don't complete high school. This is not a reflection of their righteousness.

And pain is not necessarily because of a specific defect. Remember what the Rav said? "We ask neither about the cause of evil nor about its purpose, but rather about how it might be mended and elevated." Don't worry about possible causes of evil; worry about what you can learn from it.

On the other hand, the principle of reward and punishment means that a person cannot ignore the possibility that God did intervene in this situation. If you know you have a defect, and this suffering sharpens your awareness of it, by all means, reflect on your mistake and correct it.

The point is, it's not that simple. We can know for sure that the conclusion *if I'm good, God will give me what I want, and if I'm bad, He won't*, is not true. Your spiritual level or lack thereof is not indicated by your infertility. Inability to have children is not necessarily a reflection of righteousness.

So far, Sarah seems to be taking a more practical than spiritual approach to her infertility. Let's take a look at her spiritual strategy.

---

[1] Earlier, God tells Abraham this in Genesis 12:2 and Genesis 12:7: "To your seed I will give this land," but they don't really discuss it until the aforementioned covenant.

[2] Sotah 10a

[3] Ibn Ezra (twelfth-century commentator) concurs as per Samuel II 7:11: "God will establish a house (dynasty) for you."

[4] Of course, the premise of that is that human life is valuable, which must be established before positing that anything that saves lives is valuable.

[5] What is the purpose? Is there a purpose? That question will have its own chapter later.

[6] Conclusion of a recent BusinessWeek study, paraphrased by Moshe Kranc in *The Hasidic Masters' Guide to Management*.

[7] Women seem to be more inclined to adopt or have a child with half the couple's genetic material. The maternal urge to mother a baby, *any* baby, is strong. Men tend to want a baby with *their* genetic material. I know—this is a sweeping generalization that may not apply to everyone.

[8] Samson Raphael Hirsch, *Pentateuch Translation and Commentary, Volume One: Genesis*.
[9] Adele Faber and Elaine Mazlish, *Siblings Without Rivalry*. See Chapter 2 for insight into how this multiple wife situation relates to sibling rivalry.

[10] Maimonides, Laws of Marriage 14:3.

[11] The whole interaction, found in Genesis 16:5-6, is enigmatic and requires interpretation to understand it.

[12] Page 158.

Chapter IV

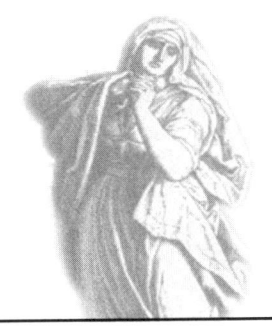

The Journey and Divine Intervention

The Spiritual Journey

Some definition of words is in order, starting with "spiritual." It has all sorts of connotations, so I want to state how I'll be using it.

Spirituality

Maimonides says that you merit eternal existence[1] based on the greatness of your deeds and the extent of your knowledge.[2] So all things that have to do with gaining the kind of knowledge that really affects you, really changes your perspective and thoughts and, ultimately, your actions, are spiritual things.

Notice that I made a leap there. Maimonides seems to say there are two separate, yet equally important factors. Deeds and knowledge. I, on the other hand, made it into one thing—the kind of knowledge that affects your deeds.

The thing that jumps out at me about Maimonides' formulation is the knowledge angle. Why do you need knowledge to get into heaven? Knowledge of what? Just be a good person. You know, do good deeds and you'll be fine.

Judaism puts a tremendous store in knowledge, but not just any kind of knowledge. There is an argument in the Talmud (Kiddushin 40b): "Which is more significant, learning or action?" The Talmud concludes: "Learning, because learning leads to action."

Hey, wait a minute. If learning is more important because it leads to action, doesn't that make *action* more important? So then why isn't the answer, "action"?

They are dependent on each other. Action without understanding doesn't cut it. Understanding without action doesn't make the grade, either.

Why not?

Action Without Understanding

Going through meaningless activities doesn't have an effect on me and doesn't reflect my inner state. Let's say I'm standing in the street and a beggar comes over to me while I'm eating my sandwich. My mother says to me, "Give him some of your sandwich." I do. This action says nothing about my compassion, my understanding of the value of human beings, my understanding of the purpose and value of charity...

Although there was a benefit in my action—the beggar got food—the action didn't really reflect *me*. The Torah values the effect on the society *and* on the individual.

The more knowledge is behind my action, the more significant it is. If I have thought deeply about how I feel about earning my own money, and what effect it has on me to give some of that money to someone in need, and why it would be worthwhile to give away money that *I* made to someone else, and what that says about me as a person and about my understanding of the world around me, and how that activity changes my perspective—

Then that action is a different action than if, never having thought about it, I gave some money to charity.

Do you see what I mean?

Understanding Without Action

It's easy to sit in an ivory tower and reflect on ideals. The challenge is in putting them to the test in the field. For example, I know that patience is important. I understand why it's important, and that being impatient is a character defect that reflects a misunderstanding of my place in the universe.

But if learning that doesn't lead to action then it isn't true learning. When I'm in traffic for forty-five minutes and someone cuts me off, if I produce a mouthful of epithets and a series of rude hand gestures, then I don't really understand the importance of patience, do I?

So the greatness of my deeds and the extent of my knowledge are not really two separate things. The greatness of my deeds reflects the extent of my knowledge. My knowledge makes my deeds great.

Back to the Journey

So Maimonides says that you merit eternal existence based on the greatness of your deeds and the extent of your knowledge. Therefore all things that have to do with gaining the kind of knowledge that really affects you, really changes your perspective and thoughts and, ultimately, your actions, are spiritual things.

Recall that in the chapter on how the Matriarchs coped with infertility, we began discussing a technique to bring about divine intervention. (Wouldn't it be great if we can get a handle on that? Remember God's warning in Isaiah: *my thoughts are not your thoughts.*)

We made the following inroad: if you want to merit divine intervention, you have to change yourself into a different person. Now, following our definition of "spiritual," we know what kind of a different person: a person with greater knowledge that expresses itself in action.

Here is an example. My father, who had a Type A personality, had expectations from his children. He wanted us to achieve. He cared about the life decisions we made, especially those that affected our potential financial success. He couldn't understand it when we had difficulty doing our homework or how we could have forgotten our books in school the night before a test.

You may have noticed that I wrote all that in the past tense. Something changed my father. When I was eighteen years old, studying in Israel for the year, my parents called me on the phone. They were on different extensions.

"Should we tell her the news?" my dad said.

"Let her guess," said my mom.

"Um..." I tried to think of the most outrageous news possible. "You're pregnant."

"That's right!"

"What?!" I said.

Anyway, we were all very excited. In May, when I came home, my baby sister was four days old. I went with my parents to a doctor's appointment the next day.

She went into the hospital the day after that. She had severe heart defects, and needed several surgeries. For the next three years, my parents were in and out of the hospital with her.

"When I found out that she might not live, I just wanted my mommy," my father said later. "Not my mother as she was then, even though I counted on her support. I mean I just wanted to be a little boy again whose mommy could make everything all better."

My father is different now. "I can't control what happens to my kids," he says. My nineteen-year-old brother wants to move to Israel and join the army instead of going to college. "It's his life—I hope he's happy," he says. My sister wants to marry a guy who hasn't finished college. He shrugs. "I hope she's happy." Any one of us makes the kind of decision that used to infuriate him and induce him to spend hours attempting to talk us out of it? His answer: "It's your life—I hope you're happy."

My father's realization that he had no control over his child's fate had a powerful impact on him. He realized that his vehement desire to control his children's lives and fates was an impotent attempt to assert control over the universe, control that he doesn't have and never will. This knowledge has changed his actions.

There is a reasonable, calmer way to talk to your kids about decisions they make. But when it comes down to it, the only life you can make decisions for is your own. My father knows that now.

All pain opens the door for potential knowledge. Let's step through the doorway.

People are Afraid of Change

When I was in high school, I was on the student council. One of the jobs of the student council was to represent the school at Open House, where you answered questions from a student's perspective.

My high school took the spiritual development of its students quite seriously. The comprehensive four-year curriculum on Spirituality came complete with extra-curricular activities, notably *Middos Tovos* nights, mandatory evening activities held four times a year that were devoted to Good Character Traits. The term is not directly translatable; it means a combination of good deeds, fine character, willingness to help others, and compassion for your fellow man.

Anyway, before Open House, the principal was giving us some pointers on how to speak to the parents and the prospective students. We were sitting in her office, looking at her across her desk. I remember it as if it were last week.

"Don't tell people that you've *changed*," she said. "People are afraid of change. They like how they are now. They don't want to think of themselves becoming different." She looked at each of us. "Use the word *growth*. Growth is good. People like to grow. They don't like to change."

Passive, Active, and Proactive in the Face of Pain

A passive person suffers and doesn't change. An active person confronts the suffering and doesn't flinch from the truths the suffering conveys. Sarah was proactive, as we'll soon see.

I want to take a moment to discuss some "existential" points. You may be wondering why this book is so philosophical. Why don't I just summarize the Matriarchs and what they did? Why do I keep talking about the universe, knowledge, understanding, and insight? Why am I talking about realizations and the changes you can make in your life? And I tell you now, we're just getting started.

I'm addressing these issues because being in pain brings up philosophical, existential questions. Why me? What is this for? What is the point of all this?

These are not fluffy questions, and don't deserve to be put off.

The fact is, if you're in pain, you're a philosopher. Animals don't react to pain by wondering about the meaning of it all. I repeat what I said before—we are abstract thinkers. No matter how much we may avoid these thoughts in our day-to-day life, there is nothing like pain to make a person start wondering.

And there is nothing like pain to put a person into a state where priorities suddenly become clearer.

Pain can lead to uncomfortable, awkward, wish-I-never-thought-about-it insight. You may have to confront motives you wish you didn't have, thoughts you would prefer to believe are beneath you, and truths that you would rather spend your life denying.

And you can. You can spend your life denying them. You can ignore your motives and your thoughts.

Or you can choose the path of the Matriarchs, and bravely face what's inside yourself and what the universe is trying to tell you.

This path brings up questions, one in particular. Okay, let's say I go through this process, and I become a really great person, way better than I am now, and I still don't get pregnant: why? Let's say I learn day and night and am very charitable: what then? Why do some people (read *me*) have to go through a process and gain insight and become a different person, which may or may not lead to results, when there are all these *other* people who seem to get pregnant with no difficulty? *Why me!*

I asked myself that question quite a few times over the years. I'm asking it here because you can't talk about gaining insight through pain without wondering why you were the lucky (read *unlucky*) person who's going through it when so many other people aren't. This is an important question and we'll come back to it later.

Now, let's look at jealousy. A major aspect of infertility is the jealousy we feel towards those who have what we want. Alone, in your house, you're okay. At work, you manage. But how many times have you burst into tears after speaking to a friend who just found out she was pregnant? Or after seeing some stranger tuck a blanket around her sleeping infant? Or after socializing with people who were all either talking about their kids or interacting with them?

What does jealousy have to show us about ourselves and the universe?

The Proactive Approach: Stimulating Potential

According to some commentaries, Sarah took active steps to change her infertility. When she gave Hagar to Abraham, she was trying to change her own childless situation, not via surrogate motherhood, but via herself becoming able to give birth to a child.

How? How can giving your husband another wife get *you* pregnant?

As we said, if you want to merit divine intervention, you must change yourself into a different person. Rashi and Sforno, two commentators, explain how it works.

Rashi comments on the effect of the words *I will be built up through her* (Genesis 16:2): "In the merit that I brought my adversary [second wife] into my house."

Sarah hopes to merit having children because she gave Hagar to Abraham. How does that follow? Bringing another woman into your house will make you worthy of being pregnant?

Sforno gives us a little more to work with. *Maybe I will be built up through her*: "Maybe the jealousy will arouse the potential into action."

According to these commentators, Sarah deliberately threw herself into a situation of jealousy on the chance that she would be able to grow from it. Generally speaking, we wouldn't choose that approach, but Sarah was relying on prophecy when she made the decision to deliberately put herself in pain (as Rashi observes in Genesis 16:2), and even then she knew that the method was not foolproof: "*Maybe I will be built up from her.*"

Sarah's actions raise some questions:

Question one: how does being jealous make you into a better person? Most of us become petty, vicious creatures when we get jealous. Jealousy usually brings out the worst in us, not the best. What potential? What action?

Question two: how does this apply to us today? We won't be bringing another wife into the household. Does the idea still relate?

There are a few approaches we can explore.

The first possibility is that the pain of the jealousy would cause Sarah to be more motivated to turn to God in prayer. We'll study exactly how that works in the chapter on Hannah. Hannah's co-wife, ahem, *adversary* Penina tried to employ the tactic of jealousy with disastrous and yet successful results. Stay tuned…

Jealousy as a Technique for Character Refinement

Another approach is that jealousy may arouse certain slumbering thoughts. Once these thoughts become conscious, you can sift through them and sort them out.

What do I mean?

Your husband has a child with another woman. That's *your* husband, *your* position, and that child should be *your* child. That should be *me*, you think. That should be *my* belly growing round with child. That should be *my* morning sickness, *my* awkwardness getting out of a chair, *my* cravings, *my baby!*

Earlier, we talked about how a human being has the ability to think about his feelings. In a situation of jealousy, there is a surge of powerful feelings. Their increased intensity makes them easier to identify. Once you've identified them, you can think about them.

One of the most important questions you can ask when you have a feeling, let's say one of hopelessness, is, "Is it true?"

You don't have to ask, "Is the feeling true? Is it true that I feel like it's hopeless?" Every feeling you have is true; it's obviously true that you feel that way. The question "Is it true?" in our example means "Is it *really* hopeless?"

I'm not trying to talk us out of our feelings. I'm not trying to make the feelings go away. I'm just trying to sort through them, sift through them, and sort of label them. Some feelings I have bring me to true conclusions; they conform to what is going on around me. But some feelings I have are not true, in the sense that they don't match what is actually happening.

Jealousy is a perfect example. I look at a woman carrying my husband's baby. I feel jealous. I feel as though that *should* be me.

But why *should* that be me? Because I *want* it to be? When did I take charge of the universe? Is it true that when I want things, they must happen? Let's look at the facts. Someone else is pregnant. Clearly, at this moment, the way the world is running, I am not pregnant. So on what basis have I determined that the world *should* be a way that it's not?

An underlying mistake in human beings' reasoning often causes jealousy. The mistake is: since I see it happening to someone in my situation, I deduce that it should happen to me, too.

Wrong. People's situations may *appear* similar, but the fact is that we each have our own unique situation. Just because the Joneses can afford a nice house, a fancy vacation and two fancy cars doesn't mean I can, too. I may have to choose. I may not have any of those options at all.

Any time I'm jealous, I can assume I'm looking at the universe through distorted eyes. Since the feelings are strong, I can become aware of them easily. And I can use the opportunity to notice where I'm making a mistake in my assumptions about my life and how it should be running.

We asked a question before: how does jealousy refine character? Usually it brings out the worst, not the best, in us. Note that jealousy does not automatically make you into a more enlightened person (wouldn't that be nice!). In fact, as per our original assessment, jealousy does indeed make you bitter and vindictive. However, understanding the root misconception that causes jealousy can give us something to think about as we're giving expectant mothers the evil eye. Realizing that we are jealous and realizing what that says about our expectations from the universe can change our perspective.

Let's take a deep breath and let that sink in before we move on to the next approach. I want us to think seriously about how we feel when we see those women parading around with their strollers or their proud bellies (or both!). I want us to think seriously about what those feelings say about how we're viewing the universe. I think this reflection is so important that I suggest you close the book, or lay it face down for a while, and think about this. You can read the rest later.

Jealousy: The Stimulus for Growth

So far we saw that we can use jealousy to give us a clearer perspective on how the universe works. If I may quote myself, "understanding how life works is the key to navigating through it with success." Recognizing what is a realistic possibility and what isn't. Maybe getting pregnant for you really *is* a realistic possibility. But if your unconscious thought is "I should have something if *they* get to have it," that's faulty reasoning. That's not how it works.

Well, that's a summary of this point. But we're not done with jealousy yet. It has more to teach us. (Never thought such a nasty emotion would be such a valuable tool, did you?)

Jealousy as a Method of Sifting between Personal and Objective Motivations

We talked earlier about *personal* versus *objective* as related to value. Let's take this discussion a little further.

When you look at them carefully, *all* motivations are actually personal. That's the way we are designed. I want something. *I* want it. So it's personal. *I* may want world peace, but if *I* want it, then it's personal. To paraphrase a popular saying: "There are no altruists in a foxhole?"[3] Actually, altruism is being *truly* selfish. You want an ideal because you think it's truly good for you. As Proverbs (11:17) says, "A kind man takes care of himself." So neither I nor the Bible is suggesting that there is any benefit in trying to do things that are not in your best interest.

If that's the case, how can jealousy help us out?

As I said before, jealousy brings up certain thoughts. Those thoughts then become accessible to you so you can examine them.

I see my husband with another wife. *That should be me.*

I see that woman pregnant. *That should be me.*

I see that woman nursing. I should get to nurse. I should get to hold my child. I should get to rock my child. I should get to sing to my child, feel its warm body against my skin, feel its tiny fingers curl around mine, look at its delicate eyelashes.

Now that I know how I feel, I can move onward to reflect on the feelings.

When I think about these feelings, I notice that my goal is largely personal satisfaction. To feel what it is to hold my own baby, to have something to love—whatever my own personal motivations are for having a baby.

As I said before, there's nothing wrong with personal motivation. As a woman, I have a powerful maternal instinct and having it gratified is very satisfying. That's our nature and that's what makes the world go 'round.

But—

Just because I want something is not a reason for me to get it. That's a childish way of thinking. I want it! I stamp my foot at the universe. So give it to me!

Think about that for a moment. Does the universe have any obligation to comply with your demand?

Of course not. Your wanting has nothing to do with getting. If you *want* a job, go to college or start sending out resumes. Don't stand there with your eyes closed, expecting it.

Previously, jealousy showed us we are making a mistake if we think that the fact that other people have something means that I should have it, too. Now, jealousy reveals another mistake in reasoning: *I want, therefore, I should get.*

Personal and Objective

As you start noticing your feelings, you will begin to see that they fit into categories. We can sort our motivations into two categories: *personal* and *objective*.

When someone says, "Put aside your personal feelings," they don't really mean for you to do something that you don't want to do. They mean for you to control yourself in one area because it will help achieve your goals in a larger framework. Achieving your goals in a larger framework is definitely not putting aside your personal feelings. It is *satisfying* your personal feelings in the broadest sense possible.

My boss did something rude to me. I fantasize about revenge. However, I put aside my *personal* desire for revenge because it will interfere with my larger desire to make a living. In this same way, I can sort my desires into ones that are purely about emotional satisfaction (hugging my sweet-smelling newborn) and ones that achieve some additional purpose.

Hold it a minute. What's the difference between gratifying a purely emotional desire and achieving a purpose? Who cares if having a baby gives me emotional satisfaction or if it continues the species? Don't I only want to continue the species out of some *emotional desire* for immortality?

There is actually a huge difference between emotional gratification and achieving a purpose. It is the difference between frustration and success. The world has a specific design. Trying to get around the design is a recipe for disappointment. If your desires coincide with the world's design, you will be successful. If your desires oppose the design, they cannot be satisfied. I may want very, very powerfully not to be subject to gravity. And I can fulfill that wish—but only if I go into outer space. As long as I'm on earth, I will be frustrated.

So I can have my personal desires, and I can try to satisfy them, under one condition: that they are in accord with the way the world works.

I can sort my desires into which ones have to do with the way the world works, and which ones want gratification that may or may not oppose the way the world works. (*I want a baby. The way the world appears to work right now, I am infertile. I don't care. I still want a baby. The universe should change to give me what I want.*)

Wanting things that achieve a purpose that the world is designed to achieve has a chance of success.

How? Having children to perpetuate the species is the way the world is designed. If I want children because I want someone to love and someone to love me, do I have less of a chance to have children than if

I want to perpetuate the species? That doesn't make sense. What do my motivations have to do with the results?

If I want to defy gravity because I think it will be fun, or if I want to defy gravity because mankind is about to be destroyed (plug in your own sci-fi plot here) and defying gravity is the only way to save the species, what's the difference? I still can't defy gravity.

That's where divine intervention comes in.

Divine Intervention
How Does This Sorting of My Thoughts Change Me and Effectuate Divine Intervention?

A word about effectuating divine intervention: this is not the sort of thing one can study scientifically. We can't take a sample of infertile women, have them apply these methods, and see if the resulting pregnancies are statistically significant.

Now, don't roll your eyes at me. (Although I admit that the scientist in me is rolling my eyes at myself. *The classic religious line*, my scientist self mocks. *I promise it works, it just can't be tested*.) Okay, go ahead. Roll your eyes at me. But let me explain what I mean.

Since, as I've mentioned, we can't really get inside God's (so-to-speak) "head," God may have other plans that do not include me getting what I want. So even if I go through all this sorting of motives and realizations about the universe, I may still be doomed to infertility. Not a particularly pleasant thought, but that is how it works. You may make some real progress and be a very different person, yet remain infertile. Remember, Hagar made a mistake when she inferred from her pregnancy some statement about her and Sarah's relative spiritual conditions.

Also, there has to be genuine realization and true change to merit divine intervention. And since only you (and sometimes not even you) and God know if that has happened, we can't make a scientific study on your secret, hidden thoughts.

What kind of a book is this, about a method that might not even work?

Our Matriarchs indicate a technique. The technique is to sort motivations into ones that solely satisfy me, and ones that match the way the universe is designed. Applying this technique is our best chance for success. If the technique fails, at least we have a fuller understanding of the way the universe is designed and our place in it. Since Man has abstract capabilities, getting a fuller understanding of something does bring its own pleasure.

Why does this technique work?

Getting in touch with motivations that coincide with the design of the universe is your best shot at meriting divine intervention.

Think of it this way. I'm running a company. The company designs...I don't know, chairs. You are my employee. You have some requests that you want me to agree to. As a reasonable employer, any of your requests that have to do with furthering my company's goal will be granted.

You want to take a class on ergonomics to learn how to apply it to chair design. Great; I'll pay for the class and let you leave work early twice a week to attend it. You want coffee breaks scheduled in so that you can discuss chair-making techniques with the other employees in a creative environment. Good idea—do you want crullers or jelly donuts? You want expensive cedar wood so that you can make higher quality chairs. You've even found a supplier. You got it. You want a two-week vacation because you're burnt out and want to come back a more productive, happier employee. Have a great time.

You want the company to supply you with a red vintage Corvette so that you can stay out late, go to parties, get smashed, and come to work late? I understand that you want that. I expect you to understand why I won't help you out with it. I'm not judging or condemning your want. Want whatever you want. Just don't expect my help if it's counter-productive to my purpose; your own personal satisfaction is not one of my goals. Your own personal satisfaction in the framework of the goals of my company is something I'm willing to help you out with. I'm not opposed to your pursuit of your own happiness; in fact I like happy employees.

To apply this little parable (that sounds so biblical, doesn't it?), the world is God's company. He designed Man with a specific nature. If we want to oppose this nature, we can go ahead. There's free will, baby. For example, people are designed to be social creatures. If you choose to be solitary, then you will suffer the consequences of loneliness. But if you want to pursue activities and values that can't satisfy you being because they clash with the way God designed humans, knock yourself out. Just don't expect divine intervention.

Ethics of Our Fathers, a work written around 200 A.D., sums it up nicely (2:4):

> "Make His will your will, so that He will make your will His will."

Tying Up Some Loose Ends

I'd just like to gather my thoughts a bit after those last few points.

What I am saying is that an infertile woman is often thrown into a situation of jealousy, and she can deal with it in a way that can lead to a greater understanding of herself and the universe. This may, through divine intervention, take care of infertility. Of course I do not know how practical the advice is in terms of divine intervention—even Sarah was only able to say "maybe." (Genesis 16:2.)[4]

An interesting point about Sarah's situation is that she really was giving up everything. There was no ruse involved; she did not secretly think that she would later cajole God into turning everything around for her, figuratively looking over her shoulder, waiting for the good times to roll in. Otherwise she wouldn't have really benefited; there would not have been any character refinement in the experience. Sarah really believed that physical continuation of Abraham's line was more important than her exclusive relationship with him. She knew the difficulties involved when she made her decision.

---

[1] What is eternal existence? That needs to be defined, too.
[2] Maimonides, *Laws of Repentance* 9:1.
[3] The real saying is a little different—some poetic license, if you will.
[4] Thanks to Maxim Khesin for this clarification.

Chapter V

Rebecca

The second Matriarch is Rebecca, or Rivka in the original Hebrew. Rebecca was infertile for a whopping twenty years. We normally don't think of Rebecca as having suffered from infertility; it's only when you do the math that this fact comes home to you.

"Isaac (*Yitzchak*) was forty years old when he took Rebecca (*Rivka*) the daughter of Besuel the Aramean from Padan Aram, the sister of Lavan the Aramean, to him as a wife." (Genesis 25:20.) Got that? Isaac was forty. "Isaac was sixty years old when she gave birth to them [Jacob and Esau]." (Genesis 25:26.)

Okay, not quite twenty years if you count the nine months of pregnancy. Plus, although the Torah doesn't give her exact age of marriage, we know that Rebecca was a young girl when she got married. Her nurse went with her. (Genesis 24:59.) It's even possible that she was married before she hit puberty.

Regardless, over a decade is a long time.

It's very interesting how the Torah expresses it. The twenty years of waiting, hoping, yearning—that whole process is condensed into *one verse*! They got married, Rebecca was barren, Rebecca conceived. As if she only took the length of time of one verse to conceive, not twenty years.

When you read it carefully, there is a lot jam-packed into this one verse, "And Isaac entreated God opposite/regarding[1] his wife, because she was barren. And God was entreated by him (i.e., accepted the prayer) and his wife Rebecca became pregnant." (Genesis 25:21.)

It appears that the primary tool used by Rebecca, Matriarch #2, is prayer. Although the plain meaning of the verse is that Isaac was the one praying, Chazal comment on the words *opposite his wife*: "One stood in one corner and prayed, and the other stood in the other corner and prayed."[2]

As I have mentioned, I plan to discuss prayer at length in the chapters about Hannah. However, we have here an introduction to prayer. Verse 21 gives us five important steps of the process: first, the activity of prayer ("And Isaac entreated God"); second, regarding/opposite; third, a cause of prayer ("because she was barren"); fourth, the acceptance of prayer ("And God was entreated by him"); and finally, a result ("and his wife Rebecca became pregnant").

Why does the verse mention that Isaac prayed opposite his wife? Does it make a difference where his wife was while he was praying? Does this teach us something about prayer?

A Husband's Longing

One thing we do see is Isaac's desire for his wife to have a child. In Genesis 21:12, God promises Abraham that it will be through Isaac that the nation will continue: "For through Isaac will offspring be considered yours." The promise is with regard to Isaac, not Rebecca. We see that Isaac entreated "regarding his wife;" he especially wanted *his wife* to be the mother of the child that would continue the mission that his parents, Abraham and Sarah, had started.[3]

To understand the other subtlety in the verse, that he entreated "opposite his wife," we have to understand what prayer is and how it works. Tune in to the chapters on Hannah. In the meantime, the Bible gives us an inside look at Rebecca's pregnancy.

Rebecca's Pregnancy

The Bible doesn't often provide details we might like to know. How did the Matriarchs carry, when they finally did get pregnant? All in front, like a watermelon, or evenly distributed? Were they blondes? Brunettes? Tall and graceful? Petite?

But we do get a peek at Rebecca's pregnancy. Genesis 25:22 tells us, "And the children banged inside her, and she said, 'If this is the case, why am I thus?' And she went to inquire of God."

Talk about ambiguous phrases.

The commentators seem to agree that Rebecca had unusual sensations during her pregnancy. Ibn Ezra says she asked around of all the local mothers and pregnant women whether they had encountered that sort of wild kicking. When she realized that she was having an unusual pregnancy, she inquired of God by consulting a prophet to find out what was going on.

Ramban says that "inquiring of God" means to pray, and that God told her (through prophecy, I assume) that she was carrying twins, which is why her pregnancy was unusual.

So far so good. Here's the tricky part. Ibn Ezra and Ramban give perfectly plausible explanations for the verse. Despite that, Rashi, Sforno, and even Ramban hint at something that is so difficult to understand, I hesitate to bring it up.

Rashi: *And she said, "If so"* – The intense pain of pregnancy. *"Why am I thus!* – Why did I desperately want and pray for pregnancy?

Sforno: *And she said, "If so"* – When they were banging and there was a fear that one of them would die and I would be at risk during the birth, as happens when delivering a still birth... *"Why am I thus!"* – Why did my relatives desire so strongly that I would have the nation's children and why did my husband pray for this?

And the crowning glory, Ramban: And she said, "*If so* – If this is the way it is going to be for me, why am I in the world? If only I didn't exist, that I would die or never have existed.

This is absolutely incomprehensible to me. Twenty years of praying, wanting, yearning, begging and entreating. It finally happens. And as we've said, Rebecca's giving birth would bring more than personal satisfaction alone. These people had a global aim—to establish a nation that would diffuse certain concepts to humanity.

I've seen it in the movies a hundred times. A good guy is shot. He needs to get the bullet out. There are no medical supplies, no painkillers, no anesthesia. His buddy sterilizes the fork they used at dinner and proceeds to dig out the bullet.

Does the shot good guy wish he had never been born? Is he sorry that the operation is happening, even though he begged his hesitant partner to do it? No! He sits there stoically during the operation. The camera zooms in for a close-up: he's in pain, teeth gritted, but he remains focused on the goal—getting that bullet out.

Are you telling me that Rebecca didn't have that same sense of clarity about her goals? That the pain made her *regret* what she was doing? It doesn't make sense. It may have been agonizing, but she would still have achieved her goals, and weren't her goals worth some pain?

Now if it were *me*, as opposed to someone with a clear understanding of her priorities like Rebecca, I could understand saying something like what Rebecca said.

The "I'm Sorry I Ever Wanted This" Mentality

We want things, but we aren't willing to take them on their own terms. For instance, part of the package of being a thief is the risk of getting caught. Part of the package of adultery is that your spouse might leave you and your kids lose respect for you. Part of drunk driving is that you can kill someone. Part of smoking five packs a day is that you risk getting lung cancer.

We don't look at things that way. In our minds, we separate the pleasure of an activity from its risks. We do what we please, and don't think about the risks being an *inseparable* aspect of our behavior. Then, if we do get stuck with the consequence, we're shocked, surprised, stunned. "I can't believe this happened," we shake our heads in wonder. "I can't believe this happened *to me*. Sure, I knew there was a risk of lung cancer. I just never thought it would happen *to me*."

Maimonides talks about the impossibility of pure pleasure in this existence.[4] There is no "good" that doesn't have "bad" with it. Everything is a trade-off. The emotional intimacy of monogamy requires the trade-off of forgoing the excitement of a variety of partners. Becoming an accomplished musician takes hours of practice.

Calculating the trade-off will reduce the shock when we encounter pain. But people don't like to think in terms of trade-offs. We like to imagine only the positives. When I'm working for an overbearing boss, I daydream about how great it would be if I owned my own business—the freedom, the creativity, the enjoyment. But when I'm self-employed, I daydream about the security of a regular paycheck. In the first case, I ignore the stress of not having a steady income. In the second, I forget the downside of serving someone else.

This whole issue came to mind when I read that Rashi commentary. When confronted with the intense pain of a difficult pregnancy, the next thought might be: "Why did I want this so badly?" You only thought about the pride you'd feel as you parade your round belly down the street. You didn't think about the incredible nausea and sleepless nights where your back aches and your belly takes up the whole bed and you toss and turn in a futile attempt to get comfortable.

Take that one step further. When you think about cradling a talcum-scented newborn, you don't imagine the frustration of being unable to ease its colicky screams at 2 AM or 3 AM or 4 AM. You don't imagine how often you'll be grouchy, tired, pushed to your limit, but still have to keep going—demanded at, cried at, with hours left to the job though your brain pleads for a break.

"I don't need to hear this," you're thinking. "I don't have a baby and I can't have one so shut up about how much pain it entails. I'd a million, billion, trillion times rather endure all that pain than the pain I'm in now!"

I know you would. So would I.

Harping on the Subject

My friend called me on the phone. "I saw a woman today with eight children. *Eight* children!" I could hear the envy dripping off the number eight. She went on to tell me how grouchy this woman was. How she snapped at her kids. How her mouth was in a tight line, her teeth clenched. How she didn't smile once at any of those eight precious souls. The implication came through loud and clear. *If those were my children, I would be smiling at them. I would cherish every beautiful moment. How can anyone act like that? This mother does not appreciate her children.*

I'm not condoning snapping at children, especially since snapping has a subtle dulling effect on children.

I was in a different situation than my friend. Although we had both been infertile for the same number of years, I was experiencing secondary infertility, trying to get pregnant again after having already had a successful pregnancy, while she had no children.

Some days, when I was struggling to manage with my whining, screaming four-year-old, I wondered, "What's wrong with me? How can I want another child when I can barely handle the one I have? Why don't I worry about not messing this one up, instead of complaining that I can't have another?"

I think it's a mistake for any of us to imagine that if (God willing, when) we finally succeed in giving birth to a first or additional child, we will never have a hard day, that we will never snap at our kids, and that the memory of the desperate yearning we feel when we are struggling to get pregnant will carry us through the day-to-day drudgery of raising children without ever resenting it. It's not realistic to believe that for the eighteen years after you conceive, you will be moved to give thanks each and every day in appreciation of the gift of a child; that when that kid lies at your feet in the supermarket screaming for candy, or speaks to you disrespectfully, you will think to yourself, "I'm so blessed." I couldn't even do that, despite the fact that I wanted a second so desperately, when I was lucky enough to have a child right there.

Maybe this is not the forum for this discussion. This is a book on infertility, and maybe it's cruel to point out that you won't appreciate your child at every moment, if and when you finally have one.

But just maybe, some of the pain of infertility is the idyllic fantasy of how the child will be. And maybe gaining a more realistic perspective on our yearning for a child would be helpful.

In the meantime, getting back to Rebecca, I don't think that the pain caused her to regret all of the effort she put in to have a child. Imagine yourself. Do you think you would regret it? So why would we expect less from our Matriarch Rebecca?

An Explanation of Rebecca's Regret

I think we have to posit what Sforno does—that Rebecca thought her life was in danger. If she were to die in childbirth, then her real goal would have been thwarted. Her goal was not to merely *have* a baby, but to *raise* that child in an atmosphere of awareness of the reality of a Creator; to educate that child so that he would have the capacity to understand the abstraction of the universe and its design without imagining multiple deities to explain the forces he observed—and to contribute another building-block in the "house" of Abraham and Sarah.

That is not achieved merely by giving birth to a child. Genes are nice. But Rebecca wanted to nurture, not just to provide nature, explains Rabbi Pelcovitz, who translated Sforno's commentary. She wanted to have Isaac's children, but not at the expense of her own life. "She had no objection to his taking another wife, as did his father, and to build his family with her."[5]

In this light, I think we can understand even the shocking sentiment that the Ramban attributes to Rebecca: "If only I didn't exist, that I would die or never have existed." Why would a person desire non-existence?

Rebecca was expressing that, if she did not survive her pregnancy to raise her child, she would not be fulfilling her purpose in terms of the larger "project" that she was involved in, in which case there was no reason to have existed.[6] She still had the purpose, as every individual has, of fulfilling her potential for personal growth and insight.

Here's an example. The president of the United States spends weeks in delicate negotiations with a country threatening nuclear war. After coming close to a resolution many times, the country stomps off in a huff and launches their bombs. The president has failed. He has failed to negotiate a treaty, failed to save his country, failed to prevent brutal and monumental bloodshed, and the country he was sworn to protect has ended up in a nuclear war. He may well feel at that point that his mission in life has failed, that his existence is purposeless. This feeling would not be a comment on the value of his personal life. He would be reflecting on his broader purpose.

So Rebecca felt that if she were unable to raise a child, the broader purpose of her existence would be unrealized. But God reassured her that the commotion in her belly was due to her carrying twins. There was a happy ending: Rebecca did indeed contribute significantly to the formation of the nation.

Rachel has a more tragic story. She ultimately dies in childbirth. Let's take a look.

[1] The word in Hebrew is *"l'nochach,"* which means both "regarding" and "physically opposite." It is difficult to capture in translation the many shades of meaning of the original language.

[2] I do wonder why Isaac's prayer is explicit, while Rivka's prayer is only implied.

[3] This in contrast to the cause of an argument between Jacob and his infertile wife, Rachel, as we shall see later.

[4] Laws of Repentance 8:1

[5] Rabbi Pelcovitz, *Sforno: Commentary on the Torah*, page 131.

[6] Moses expressed a similar sentiment when he was bargaining for the Jews' lives after the sin of the Golden Calf. "And now, if you would forgive their sin. And if not, please erase me from your book that you have written." (Exodus 32:32.) Radak, a twelfth-century commentator, quotes Moses' request in interpreting Jonah 4:3. It seems to indicate that when a prophet is unable to fulfill his task of helping his nation, his existence becomes meaningless. Not in a personal way, because an individual can always pursue a personal relationship with his Creator, but in a "mission-specific" way.

Chapter VI

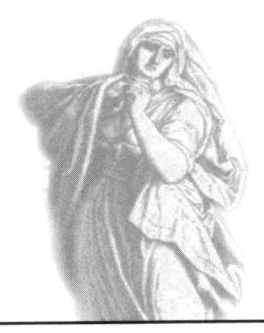

Rachel

Let's start with the usual: establish Rachel's infertility and calculate the approximate number of years she was infertile.

We've already discussed Rachel's infertility in comparison with her co-wife and sister, Leah. "And God saw that Leah was hated and he opened her womb; and Rachel was barren." (Genesis 29:31.) Between verses 32 through 35, Leah delivers four sons; assuming absolutely no spacing, 9 x 4 = 36 months. Three years of infertility so far.

Genesis 30:1-25 relates the following story:

> Rachel saw that she wasn't bearing Jacob children and she was jealous of her sister. She said to Jacob, "Give me children! And if not, I am dead." Jacob's anger flared up at Rachel, and he said, "Am I instead of God who has withheld from you fruit of the womb?" She said, "Here is my maidservant Bilhah; consort with her, and she will give birth on my knees and I will also be built up from her [*same plan as Sarah!*]." And she gave him Bilhah her maidservant as a wife, and Jacob consorted with her. Bilhah conceived and bore Jacob a son. Rachel said, "God has judged me and also heard my voice and gave me a son;" that's why she called him Dan [from the root *to judge*]. She conceived again, and Bilhah, maidservant of Rachel, bore a second son to Jacob. And Rachel said, "Struggles of God have I struggled with my sister, and I, too,

have succeeded." [This is a phrase with many connotations; I chose one.] And she named him Naftali [from the root to *struggle*, to *scheme*, to *pray*, to *tie*].

And Leah saw that she had stopped giving birth, and she took Zilpah her maidservant and gave her to Jacob as a wife. [Apparently, Leah, too, experienced some infertility, though it was secondary—she already had children; and she, like Rachel, used Sarah's method.] And Zilpah, Leah's maidservant, bore Jacob a son. And Leah said, "Good luck has come!" [also an indeterminate word] and she named him Gad. Zilpah the maidservant of Leah bore a second son to Jacob. Leah said, "In my good fortune! Because women have deemed me fortunate!" and she named him Asher [root *happy/fortunate*].

Reuven [Leah's oldest son] went in the days of the wheat harvest and he found *dudaim* [a type of plant] in the field and he brought them to Leah his mother. And Rachel said to Leah, "Please give me some of your son's *dudaim*." And she said to her, "Isn't it enough that you took my husband? And now you will also take my son's dudaim?" And Rachel said, "That's why he will sleep with you tonight in exchange for your son's dudaim." Jacob came from the field in the evening, and Leah went out to greet him and she said, "You will come to me because I have hired you with my son's dudaim." And he lay with her that night. And God listened to Leah, and she conceived and bore Jacob a fifth son. And Leah said, "God gave me my reward for giving my maidservant to my husband" [as Sarah had been hoping when she gave her husband Hagar]. And she named him Issachar [from the root to *reward*]. And Leah conceived again and bore a sixth son to Jacob. And she said, "God bestowed on me a good gift. This time my husband will dwell with me because I have borne him six sons," and she named him Zevulun [from the root to *dwell*]. Afterwards, she bore a daughter and named her Dina.

And God remembered Rachel, and God listened to her, and opened her womb. She conceived and bore a son, and she said, "God has gathered up/cut off my humiliation." And she named him Joseph [*Yosef* in Hebrew, from the root to *gather/cut off/ add*], saying "May God add on for me another son." And it was when Rachel had given birth to Joseph, Jacob said to Lavan, "Send me and I will go to my place and my land."

There is a lot of information here! Let's sort it all out.

One thing we see is that Joseph's birth coincides with the end of the seven-year payment plan. As you may recall, after Lavan tricked him into marrying Leah, Jacob agreed to work for Lavan for a second stretch of seven years so that he could marry Rachel. So altogether, Rachel was infertile for less than seven years—not as long as Sarah or Rebecca, but still quite a long time. Rachel's pain is explicitly discussed in the Bible. Let's look at an argument she had with Jacob after she had been infertile for about three years.

Rachel's Pain

"And Rachel saw that she didn't bear children for Jacob, and Rachel was jealous of her sister. And she said to Jacob, "Give me children! And if not, I am dead." (Genesis 30:1.)

People have different thresholds of tolerance for pain. There is no strict correlation between years of infertility and degree of pain. Rachel's three-year pain is recorded, while Rebecca's two decades or Sarah's lifetime of childbearing years are not. Your five years of infertility could be more painful than someone else's ten years.

According to Ramban, Rachel was asking Jacob to pray for her and to keep praying until God granted her children, no matter what. And if not, she would die of pain. Her jealousy caused her to speak inappropriately (as we'll see when we discuss Jacob's response), and she thought that Jacob would fast and don sackcloth and pray, because of his deep love for her, until she had children, so that she wouldn't die of anguish.

Ramban attributes her strong language to jealousy, and not to the anguish of infertility. As we discussed in Sarah's chapter, the two are intertwined. Rachel was not just jealous of her sister's emotional gratification at having children; Rachel wanted to participate in the building of the nation.

Another Poignant Rashi

On the words *I am dead*, Rashi comments: "From here we learn that whoever has no children is considered dead."

Hold on a second. In what sense is a childless person dead? Take any random person who has no children; let's call her Shirley. Is Shirley dead? Hardly. Does anyone consider her so? I would think not. It seems insulting to consider a childless person dead.

And just to be thorough, I'd like to know how "dead" is different than "broken." Remember that statement from Chazal's commentary about Sarah? "Whoever has no children is not built, rather, broken." Chazal don't just say things to express sentiment. They must be conveying more than "infertility is sad" or "infertility is painful."

Am I Trying to Make Us Feel Worse?

I hate to bring up these statements of Chazal. Here we are feeling miserable enough already about our own personal deprivation of not having children, and then I start talking about being broken and considered dead. Not a very comforting way of looking at things. We're only going to feel worse.

So what am I trying to do here?

Well, I personally do find it comforting to know that the Sages observe that childlessness is a real loss. In fact, I find it more than comforting; I find it helpful. The Sages are pointing out the objective loss of childlessness. Sorting the motivations that are purely personal from the ones that coincide with how the world works is the key to effectuating possible divine intervention.

And even if I never achieve divine intervention, I still want to face facts. The best way to cope with pain is to acknowledge it. If I can't admit the pain to myself, then it's always there, and I'm always avoiding it.[1] The Sages are revealing a reality about childlessness. We can't wriggle out of it.

So Why Is a Childless Person Considered Dead?

We can rule out *physically* dead. That's obvious. *Psychologically* dead? Rachel's statement does have the connotation that she will die of pain if she has no children. "Give me children! And if not, I am dead!" Okay, that's a possibility. Let's hold that thought. We can also rule out *spiritually* dead, since spirituality has to do with a person's deeds and knowledge, and is achievable without children.

I think the Sages are actually talking *socially*. A childless person is considered dead socially.[2]

I'm sure you know just what I mean. Don't you dread social situations? Why? Because everyone (all right, let's be honest—not *every*one, but it sure feels that way) in your peer group is in the process of raising children. This is a major endeavor in which human beings are engaged at this point in their lives, ages twenty through forty and beyond—decades of your having to be in social situations with people who are devoting their energy and resources to raising children. And although many people *are* able to evaluate you for who *you* are, not whom you're raising, there is a certain attitude that you encounter...

One time, when I had been trying to conceive for about a year and a half, I was at lunch with three other couples. The hostess was newly married (read "not yet expected to have kids"). The other two couples were the proud parents of infants. After lunch, the men were doing whatever, the hostess was in the kitchen, and I was trapped with two cooing new moms.

"So what are you doing about weaning?" one asked.

"Oh, she still nurses three times a day! I'm not even thinking about it yet." Pat, pat her darling baby.

"You can do it gradually by weaning off one feeding each week or so," I offered. I wasn't thrilled with the topic, but I could either participate or go to the bathroom and cry.

The mom who asked the question looked at me blankly for a moment. Then she turned to the other mother and said, "What about sleeping? Does your baby sleep through the night?" She didn't even acknowledge me!

Do I sound bitter? I was very hurt. It still hurts just thinking about it.

I'm sure you've all encountered it: the callousness, the implication that if you are not a parent, you can't possibly know anything about child-rearing; the feeling of being excluded because you're not doing what the rest of them are doing. You're out of the club. In the same way, a dead person is not really significant, not really part of life, does not have the same status as the living.

In truth, many do not consider childless people in any way inferior to people who have children. However, raising children is an accomplishment, a consuming interest, a bonding experience. And when people are doing that, we can't participate, in much the way that a dead person can't participate in life.

Rachel's situation was particularly difficult. She watched her sister Leah busily having and raising children, while she was unable to join the third generation in the mission of building the nation. Let's see how Jacob answered her.

Jacob's Rebuke – A Husband's Insensitivity?

"Jacob's anger flared up at Rachel and he said, 'Am I instead of God who has withheld from you fruit of the womb?'" (Genesis 30:2.)

Whoa, Jacob! Harsh response! "Who do you think I am, God? Is it *my* fault you're not pregnant?"

To be honest, at first glance, the commentators don't make it look better. Rashi, quoting Chazal as usual, says: "You say that I should do like my father [Isaac] [and pray for you]. I am not like my father. My father didn't have children. I have children. God prevented from you, not from me."

Ouch!

Where's the empathy? Where's the concern for his beloved wife? How can he say such a thing when she's in so much pain? This sure puts your own husband's inability to relate to your pain in perspective, doesn't it?

In fact, the Sages do comment on the seeming callousness: "Is this the way to answer a woman who is oppressed by her barrenness?" [3]

Jacob must have spoken like that for a good reason. We know that Jacob loved Rachel. The Bible tells us straight out in Genesis 29:18, 29:30, and most noticeably 29:20: "Jacob worked for Rachel for seven years, and they seemed in his eyes like a few days because of his love for her." Also, the Bible itself says, "Don't verbally oppress." (Leviticus 25:17.) Common decency should prevent you from verbally oppressing someone who is in a great deal of pain. I'm holding the Patriarch Jacob to at least that standard.

A Husband's Rebuke

Do you ever get so involved in the tragedy of your own pain, or so insular about the severity of your suffering, that you might benefit from a good slap in the face?

On the surface, Rachel wanted her righteous husband to pray on her behalf. But Jacob heard certain premises and subtle implications in her choice of words. When we look carefully at his response, and compare it to her words, we see what he was addressing.

The harsh approach was effective; it was precisely its severity that helped Rachel see that she had phrased her request inappropriately. He chose exactly the right words to clarify certain fundamental truths.

Truth #1: There Are No "Miracle Workers"

"Give me children!" Rachel demanded, as if Jacob himself had the power to do so.[4] Jacob's anger flared up. "Am I instead of God?"

Jacob reacted in anger to the implication that a human being has the power to grant something that only God can give. Human beings simply do not have that kind of power. No human being can supernaturally help an infertile woman have a child. The closest we get are infertility specialists, who employ their knowledge of science and the laws of nature to help a couple achieve fertility.

Truth #2: You Can't Make God Do What You Want

A *demand* for children makes a false statement about the nature of prayer, and, more fundamentally, the nature of Man's relationship with God.

"Am I instead of God?" Jacob said, meaning "Can I take God's place? You have to realize that I cannot force God to accept my prayer." Ramban thinks it was obvious that Jacob *was* praying for Rachel.[5] Obviously God had not granted his request. "It's in the hands of God, not in *my* hands," he was saying. "Do you think *I'm* in charge?"

Nehama Leibowitz, a modern Biblical commentator, makes a shocking statement in her commentary on this area. Any attempt to sway God to do your will with the intention of subjugating God through some means—whether you use sacrifices, dances, incantations, all sorts of mumbo jumbo, or prayer (!)—to bend to your own will, is nothing more than magic and idolatry. A true petitioner knows that his prayer *does not have the power* to force God his Creator; he knows that God is God, and will do what is good in His eyes.[6]

You hear that? It's not the action, it's the underlying attitude. The most virtuous-looking action can be nothing more than a distorted attempt to bend God to your will. And that makes it worthless.

Truth #3: It's Not About Me, It's About You

"Give me children!" Rachel said. "Am *I* the one who's preventing the fruit of your womb?" asked Jacob. "*I* have children. *You* don't."

Rachel was looking to Jacob to solve the problem. Jacob redirected her. You want *me* to give you children. It's not *me* you should be looking to, it's yourself. It's *your* relationship with God, *your* desire. This is not about me. It's about you.

Ultimately, we are each responsible for our own situation. Nobody can do it for us. Nobody can change us. Someone else praying for me will not affect me the way my own efforts can.

Truth #4: The Real Purpose of Your Existence

I think Truth #4 deserves its own chapter.

---

[1] For example, if I stoically maintain that it didn't really bother me that my sister lied to me and stole $50,000 and ran away with my husband, then I'm going to have some trouble healing.

[2] I'm basing this on another statement of the Sages: "A poor person is considered dead" (Tractate Nedarim 64b), i.e. a poor person does not have social clout.

[3] Bereshis Rabbah 71:19—Chavel's translation from Ramban's commentary on Genesis 30:2.

[4] Sforno 30:2.

[5] Genesis 30:2. In the Bible there are instances where prophets prayed for strangers; of course Jacob would pray for his own wife.

[6] Nehama Leibowitz, Studies in Bereshit (Genesis), page 232.

Chapter VII

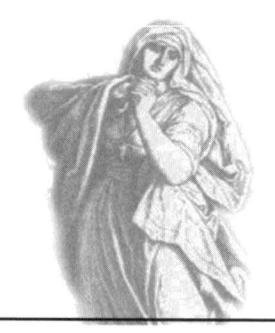

The Real Purpose of Your Existence

Perhaps you think I am being overly-dramatic to have ended the chapter there, but I honestly believe that this is the most important chapter of the book. Please give it your full attention.

Rachel was so focused on the importance of having children that she missed an important point.[1] "Give me children—and if not, I am dead!" Or, said another way, "There is no reason for me to exist if I can't have children."

Jacob grew angry at that statement, which is simply not true. It is not true that your life is meaningless if you can't have children.

Let's go back to Genesis. When we first meet Woman, she has been created from Adam's rib. In Genesis 2:23 she is called *"Isha"* (Woman) because she was taken from Man (*Ish*, in Hebrew). Jump a chapter ahead, to Genesis 3:20, and Woman is called *"Chava"* ("Eve" in English; from the Hebrew root *chai*, meaning "life") because she is the "mother of all living."

These two names indicate two purposes to Woman's life. The first purpose, the primary purpose, is to be a human being.

By "purpose" I don't mean cosmic expectation. I mean take a look at how any given object is made, look at its design, determine how it is meant to be used, and that's its purpose. Like a chair. Take a look at a chair. What is it for? Sitting. The purpose of a chair is for people to sit in it, not to wear it on their heads or carry it home full of groceries.

So the primary design of a Woman is to be a human being. You have the ability, the same as a man, to understand and advance in the intellectual and moral fields.[2]

The secondary purpose alludes to the power of childbearing and rearing children, indicated by the name "Eve," mother of all living. *Akeidas Yitzchak* calls this a Woman's *little* purpose, as opposed to her *primary* purpose of being a human being. A Woman deprived of the power of childbearing is deprived of her *little* purpose, and is left only with her primary purpose. Jacob was therefore angry with Rachel. He reprimanded her to make her understand an all-important principle—that, as far as their joint purpose in life, she is not dead just because she is childless.

Nehama Leibowitz comments on this interpretation. I think her words speak to all of us who yearn for a child:

> She in her yearnings for a child saw her whole world circumscribed by the second purpose of woman's existence (according to the Akeidas Yitzchak, "the secondary purpose"!) to become a mother. Without it, her life was not worth living. "Or else I die." This was a treasonable repudiation of her function, a flight from her destiny and purpose, shirking the duties imposed on her, not in virtue of her being a woman, but in virtue of her being a human being.[3]

Why do I believe that this is the most important chapter in this book? Because our secondary purpose, to be a mother, may sometimes feel so consuming that we forget about our primary nature—to be a human being. The maternal instinct is powerful. The urge to procreate is strong. Jacob reminded Rachel, and the record of this conversation reminds us through the generations: procreation is secondary to what you do with your own life. It is what you choose to do with your own life that is your primary purpose.

---

[1] This chapter is based on the commentary by Rabbi Yitzchak Arama (1420-1494), called *Akeidas Yitzchak*.

[2] Note that Rabbi Yitzchak Arama's understanding of the nature of human beings coincides with what we have discussed about the unique nature of Man.

[3] Leibowitz page 335.

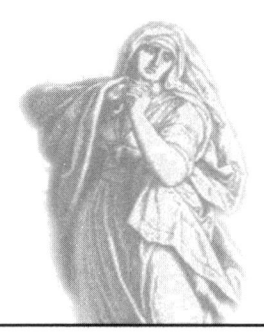

Chapter VIII

Rachel Continued

Rachel's Response

Rachel responds to Jacob's challenge. She accepts that if she is to have children, it is up to her to look within herself. Rachel does not flinch from the cold truths that Jacob has pointed out to her. To reiterate:

> She said, "Here is my maidservant Bilhah; consort with her, and she will give birth on my knees and I will also be built up from her." And she gave him Bilhah her maidservant as a wife, and Jacob consorted with her. Bilhah conceived and bore Jacob a son. Rachel said, "God has judged me and also heard my voice and gave me a son;" that's why she called him Dan [from the root *to judge*]. (Genesis 30: 3-6.)

Rachel, following the example of the Matriarch Sarah, gives her maidservant to her husband in the same hope that motivated Sarah: "I *too* will be built up from her." *Too*, in addition to Sarah. We can assume the same dual purpose as Sarah had. First, to be involved in raising and educating a child, even if it is someone else's; second, to merit having a child of her own.[1]

Note that Rachel chooses the child's name.[2] This indicates her participation in the raising of the child. (Would you let someone else name *your* child?) The names are significant and fascinating. We will be looking at some of them.

Rachel's Introspection

"God has judged (*Dan*) me, and also heard my voice and gave me a son." Through the name, Rachel describes the process and its outcome.

God has judged me. She accepts the justice of God's decree of her infertility. Sforno: "God was just in His decree that He did not give me pregnancy." She took Jacob's words to heart. This is a different sentiment than "Give me children or else I am dead!" She accepts the reality of her situation: God did not give her pregnancy.

How did she come to this conclusion? Unfortunately, we don't get a play-by-play of her internal process, but we can posit a possible outline of its general steps based on the concepts we've been discussing. First, she considers giving Jacob her maidservant. Then, as we discussed in Sarah's chapter, her jealousy highlights the feeling, "That should be me." The intensity of this feeling makes it more noticeable. Noticed feelings are the easiest to examine: have a strong feeling, notice the feeling. Noticing it allows her to examine the feeling more rationally: "Is this really true?" She arrives at her conclusion: "I accept the reality that I'm not pregnant. There is no *should*. What is, is."

Our Best Shot at Developing Effective Strategies

Rachel illustrates for us something we said earlier: "Understanding how life works is the key to navigating through it with success." Accepting a situation is the prerequisite for planning a strategy to deal with it. It is the acceptance of reality that allows a person to move forward, as Rachel did in this case. We use up all of our energy if we fight against the way things are.

Why? Because it's impossible to analyze a situation with a clear head if you're busy thinking that it shouldn't be happening. You won't be able to figure out what to do. All of your planning will be interrupted by the thought, "This shouldn't even *be* like this!" If it shouldn't be like that, then you don't have to fix it, right? Because if it shouldn't be like that, and you keep your eyes closed long enough, then it will go away. Right? Really...right?

We wish. Keep wishing. In the meantime, these sneaky little thoughts will prevent you from dealing with your situation in a useful way. The wish to have things magically go our way is so powerful that it can actually interfere with our realistic attempts to cope.

For example: I can't stand my boss. He alternates between degrading me by sending me out for coffee, and packing in tons of work but stealing the credit for himself. I spend all my free time complaining: "I don't understand what I ever did to deserve a boss like him. It's so unfair. How come other people have *normal* bosses? How come other people have some sort of job satisfaction? How come *I* have to worry every day that my psychopathic boss is going to stick me with a project due yesterday?"

Do you see where all my energy is going in this example? It isn't going toward finding solutions. It's being used to maintain the illusion that this *shouldn't be happening to me*.

Go ahead, make a list. As an objective observer, you can probably come up with multiple solutions for me right off the top of your head. Solution one: quit. Solution two: objectively evaluate the pros and cons of this job. If I decide that the pros (good salary, potential, and benefits) outweigh the cons (difficult boss), focus on the pros after making the decision to stay. Realize that it is *my* decision to stay in this job, not a quirky cosmic joke with me as the victim. Solution three: strategize about how to handle myself when my boss sends me for coffee. Would a discussion work? Going to his superior? Solution four: examine my own feelings. Why does this bother me so much? Deep down, do I agree with his implication that I'm inferior?

Why am I not thinking along any of those lines? Because I'm stuck. I'm stuck hating my situation. The way out of it is to take a cold, clear look around me, to look at my situation with the objectivity of a doctor making a diagnosis.

Diagnose, even if it's painful. Then you can begin treatment.

Back to Rachel's Plan

"God has judged me, and also heard my voice and gave me a son."

And also heard my voice. Rachel no longer despairs about her situation. She confronts it in a strong, realistic way. If the only way she can take part in building the nation is by raising someone else's child, then she is determined to do that. She prays that her plan will be successful.

I know that we still haven't discussed prayer and how it works. We'll get to it, I promise.

And gave me a son. Rachel accepts that this is her situation, this is her solution, and this is her son. She rejoices that her plan was successful and she can participate in building the nation.

Rashi quotes Chazal on *God has judged me*: "He judged me, he found me guilty, and he found me meritorious." This sums up the process. In the state she was in before, the judgment was that she would not have children. After her process of introspection and giving her maidservant to Jacob, the judgment changed. As a result of her own initiative (after a little nudge from Jacob), she was deemed worthy to bring up a child.

A Shift in Focus

Rachel's strength of character is inspiring. According to Chazal, she said, "God found me worthy." Not worthy of having her *own* child; worthy of participating in the building of the nation. She has changed focus. The person who claimed that her life was over if she couldn't have children now feels privileged to be even the mere impetus of a child! Like Sarah, she plans to find satisfaction in being the *cause of its existence and the means of its spiritual development*. We know how much pain she was in. She has changed her whole perspective. Her willingness to act from this new perspective is heroic.

The story does not end here. Let's look at the next son.

Rachel's Struggle

"She conceived again, and Bilhah, maidservant of Rachel, bore a second son to Jacob. And Rachel said, 'Struggles of (*naftulay*) God have I struggled (*niftalti*) with my sister, and I too have succeeded.' And she named him Naftali. (*Naftali* comes from the root, to *struggle*, to *scheme*, to *pray*, to *tie*)." (Genesis 30:7-8.)

Method of the Torah

These verses are a prime example of the Torah's infinite depth. This one phrase lends itself to many possible interpretations. If we follow each thread separately, it will lead us to its own treasure-trove of insight. "Your ears should listen to wisdom, and incline your heart to understanding... If you seek it like silver; search for it like hidden treasure." (Proverbs 2:2 and 2:4.) This next discussion will take us on a hunt for buried jewels. Four commentators have marked an X. Let's start digging.

Prayer

Onkelos, whose second-century Aramaic translation of the Torah is, according to the Columbia Encyclopedia, "almost as authoritative a text as the Pentateuch itself," translates the words *naftulay* and *niftalti* based on the root for prayer, *t'fila*.[3]

This "authoritative" translation says that Rachel is describing the success of her prayers. "I begged and pleaded and prayed many prayers." Two things strike me about this.

First, I find it very moving that Rachel considers a child born by another woman to be a success. "And I, too, have succeeded." She considers someone else's giving birth to have been a successful response to her prayers! Rachel's greatness really impresses me. She has so completely accepted her situation, and she so joyously describes the extent to which she *can* participate in this child's upbringing. True, she anticipates the enjoyment of raising a child, but she knows she will miss out on the egocentric gratification of bringing up a child with her *own genes* ("don't you think he has my brains?") or the intense pleasure of watching a child that is a part of *her flesh* ("he always was energetic, even when I was carrying him"). Yet she considers this child, literally, "the answer to all her prayers"—a child that is not biologically hers.

The second thing that catches my attention is the role of prayer in her success. It seems that Rachel had already attributed success to prayer when she had her first (adopted) son. Why bring it up again? After Dan's birth, Rachel emphasized her acceptance that God had "judged" her and that was the reason she was not getting pregnant. Part of the idea was that when she had accepted this, God answered her prayers for a son in her new framework. "God judged me and also heard my voice [prayer] and He gave me a son." (Genesis 30:5.) Now, with the birth of her second son, Rachel is again focusing on prayer. What's new in this second case?

Rachel is imparting how vital prayer is. She describes prayer as the essential ingredient in the birth of her second child.

You might be getting annoyed already. I keep mentioning prayer; every Matriarch employs prayer, and yet we haven't sat down and explained what exactly prayer is and how it works. When we do, though, you can go back and take a new look at all the prayer discussed in the stories of the Matriarchs. In the meantime, let's take a look at Rashi's X-marks-the-spot.

Stubbornness

According to Onkelos, Rachel proclaims this child to be a response to her prayers. Rashi agrees.[4] He does, however, add one intriguing ingredient to the mix. "I was stubborn and I"...I think the best word is *badgered*— "badgered many badgerings and schemes to God in order to be equal to my sister."

This is very strange. What is this concept of harassing God for what you want? What kind of schemes does Rashi have Rachel exulting over? I know you can't manipulate God, so what sort of process is Rachel describing here? And even weirder, whatever the process is, it seems to have worked!

Let's absorb the difficulty of this question for a moment.

There are two different flavors here. There is harassing, badgering, pressuring, urging. And there is scheming, twisting, turning, maneuvering.

We can rule out one possibility. Rachel is not trying to make God change his mind. God doesn't change. Remember? So we have to explain what Rachel is accomplishing by "badgering" God with prayer.

As we said previously, changing yourself is the only way to change your situation. Rachel is revealing an important characteristic in this arena: determination. She is giving us the key to success. You must be determined. You must be willing to continue your struggle, your attempts. You must persist.

And yet, we see another characteristic that balances the determination: adaptability. Twist and turn. You may try one approach, but it may not work. You cannot get stuck in your narrow view of how things should be. You have to maneuver. You have to twist. You have to try something else. You have to be able to adjust to new possibilities, even those you would rather not consider. You have to be able to see their potential, and make the most of them.

And here is where we see Rachel's greatness. The combination of determination and adaptability. She did not give up her desire for children—she adapted. Dan and Naftali were the successful fulfillment of her desire.

One aspect of Rachel's words bothers me: her feelings about her sister. The implication is that Rachel is struggling with, or wanting to be equal to, her sister. This doesn't quite fit the picture I have of Rachel, who is so focused on building the nation, with all of her efforts directed towards that goal. Shouldn't she be above something as petty as sibling rivalry?

Wrestling/Struggling

Ibn Ezra comes back to this point and marks a spot for us to dig. A prominent grammarian, he defines *naftal* as "wrestling with someone to be victorious over him in order to topple him." That would mean that Rachel was wrestling with Leah (metaphorically, regarding motherhood?) to be victorious over her. This interpretation does not exactly set my mind at rest.

"Struggles of God I have struggled with my sister, and I was successful." Why bring God into this? If this is about one-upping your sister, is that the kind of thing God helps us with? Ibn Ezra raises that specific point: why does it mention "God?" Because God helped me in my wrestling.

He also suggests the possibility that Rachel calls it a Godly struggle with her sister because it was for the honor of God that she gave her maidservant. This certainly doesn't seem to be about two sisters bickering and jockeying for position. Trying to topple your sister and maintaining that it's for the honor of God sounds almost delusional. We still need an explanation.

I hope your curiosity is piqued. We'll come back to this subject of Rachel's jealousy of her sister Leah.

Partnership between Two Sisters

Sforno interprets Rachel's statement about Leah in a more cooperative way. Rather than interpreting it as a struggle *against* Leah, Sforno interprets *naftal* as "bound" or "tied." Rachel is bound together with her sister Leah in their struggle to achieve a common goal.[5] They have a partnership. They are a team working together on the mission of building a nation.

When Leah stops having her own children, she follows her sister's example of employing an alternate strategy, as we will see.

Now let's make a little visit to the nursery of Rachel's long awaited first-born son.

Joseph

> Reuven went in the days of the wheat harvest, and found *dudaim* in the field, and he brought them to Leah his mother. And Rachel said to Leah, "Please give me some of the *dudaim* of your son." And Leah said, "Isn't it enough that you took my husband? And now you want to take my son's *dudaim* also?" And Rachel said, "Therefore he'll lie with you tonight in exchange for your son's *dudaim*." (Genesis 30:14-15.)

> God remembered Rachel; God hearkened to her and He opened her womb. She became pregnant and she bore a son, and she said, "God has gathered/ended [*asaf*] my humiliation." She called his name Joseph [*Yosef* in Hebrew] saying, "May God add on [*yosef*] for me another son." (Genesis 30:22-24.)

The Formula for Success

Verse 22 uses two phrases to describe how God related to Rachel. He "remembered" her and He "listened" to her. Why two? They both mean the same thing—that God intervened.[6]

Okay, true. They obviously don't mean *exactly* the same thing. Let's rephrase the question. What kind of intervention does the word "remembered" mean and what different kind of intervention does the word "listened" mean?

Ever alert to these types of subtleties, Sforno comes to our rescue. "Remembering" is a response to Rachel's *efforts* to have children. "She tried to have children by bringing her adversary into her house and with regard to the dudaim." (30:22.) Listening is different. It is a response to her prayer. "She prayed after she had done two types of efforts."

This gives us a two-pronged approach: *action* and *prayer*.

Two Categories of Action

Rachel focused her efforts in two areas. One, the handing over of her maidservant to her husband, we have discussed at length. It is a spiritual effort, designed to make a person aware of any feelings that contradict how the world actually works. The other effort was the *dudaim*.

Um, what are *dudaim*?

We can infer that they are a type of plant that grows at the time of the wheat harvest. But why did Rachel want them? What did she want to do with them, and how would they help in her effort at pregnancy?

The commentators have different opinions as to what exactly *dudaim* are. Among the possibilities: a herb that would coax conception, a male aphrodisiac, and a mood-setting perfume.

Rachel used every natural resource available. She attacked her problem with both physical and spiritual approaches.

The Action/Prayer Partnership

The recipe is action and prayer. This gives us a fascinating little reminder. No matter how much a human being tries to plan, there is a world of details that are outside of human control. Whenever we attempt anything, no matter how thorough we are, we can't cover all of them. When I'm going on a job interview, I can be well-informed, dress to look attractively professional, and have textbook interpersonal skills. But no matter how many memos I jot in my Franklin Planner, it's useless to list "Note to self: make sure interviewer is in receptive mood." That is one thing that is out of my control. Maybe the interviewer is a bear that day because his sister called him that morning, frantic that they urgently have to put their aging father in a nursing home, and his teenage son slammed out the door when Dad commented on his pierced tongue. And to top it off, the interviewee before me oozed competence and confidence. I never had a chance—and all because of a confluence of factors beyond my control.

That doesn't mean it's pointless to try. Giving up in advance is the best way to get zero results. "Gee, I'll just twiddle my thumbs and see if I can get a job that way. Hey, you never know. Crazier things have happened." But the "action plus prayer" approach shows us that we have to take our best shot, even knowing that we don't call all the shots.

Rachel's pregnancy was the result of her efforts *and* her prayer.

What's in a Name?

There's something a little puzzling about Joseph's name. Verse 24 says that she named him Yosef (from the root to *add on*) to express the hope that she would have another son. That bothers me. Why doesn't she savor the gift of this son? Already, in the delivery tent, she's looking for the next one? The essence of this son is that she should have another?

This is particularly puzzling when we consider the implication of Joseph's name from the previous verse, "God has gathered/ended (*asaf*) my humiliation." *Asaf* has the same root as *Yosef*. If the main idea of Joseph's name is that Rachel is already asking for another son, then what was the point of her more appreciative interpretation of the name in the previous verse? Is the name to call to mind the end of her humiliation or the hope for another son, or both?

Rashbam (Rashi's grandson and a commentator in his own right) says that Joseph's name is essentially to express the ending of her humiliation. The double meaning of the name just provided an opportunity to tag on a prayer for another child.

Ibn Ezra comments: "God saw the humiliations; the women used to humiliate me because I was barren."

The Humiliation of Being Childless

Humiliation is a fascinating subject. Not the experience—that's just painful. Humiliation is that sick feeling we get when we think other people are thinking negative things about us. The irony is, your worth has nothing to do with other people's opinions; they can only judge on partial evidence. Do we agree on this? Everybody knows that you can't judge a book by its cover. When nobody's looking, Mr. Pillar-of-the-community may kick a puppy that annoys him, or engage in insider trading. A socially awkward girl who wears a skirt that is the wrong color, style, or length may be scorned by her classmates though she is intelligent and kind.

And yet, as much as *logically* we know that opinion does not equal actual value, when someone thinks badly of us—it hurts. Social disapproval is one of the most intense forms of pain a human being can experience.

When people know you're having problems getting pregnant, it can be humiliating. Personally, I didn't feel embarrassed about my infertility—I'm more of a "capitalize on all the sympathetic attention" kind of gal—but I have a close friend who found it a constant source of humiliation. There is an odd shame in not having children because, as we know, there is not necessarily a correlation between a person's worth—her true value—and the results she obtains (such as pregnancy, popularity, or riches).

Here's an analogy: who is superior? A person who's missing an arm, but has strong values and lives by them? Or a person with two arms who lies, cheats and steals? The one-armed man of principle, right? Sure. We all agree. And yet, it's possible for the person with the missing arm to feel deficient, though in reality, he may be more complete.

A lot of humiliation is about insensitivity. A childless person brings out pity and gossip. People *love* to talk about the problems of others. Some people are just vicious; others disguise their glee at our misfortune as sympathy. The more we childless consider ourselves a target for gossip because of our deficiencies, the more humiliated we feel. I read the complaints on infertility website message boards—believe me, people demonstrate insensitivity to the pain of infertility in endless permutations. Someone suggested to a childless—pardon me, child-*free*—friend of mine that she and her husband get a dog. That should take care of the problem.

If we focus on our *actual* worth, separate from other people's opinions, we can turn things completely around. The things we feel embarrassed about may not really be defects, and maybe the areas we need to work on are things nobody knows about.

Another Possibility

Remember people's misinterpretation of barrenness from Hagar and Sarah? People assume that if one of the women of this illustrious family can't have children, she must not be on a high enough level to merit it. (Genesis 16:4.)

We don't know how the attitude of others affected Rachel. We can imagine how *we* would feel in her situation, but each person's sensitivities are different. Put aside for a minute any personal pain that Rachel might have felt when she noticed other people degrading her— there was another factor at work. Rachel's infertility looked bad for the mission that she and her family were involved in. The disgrace of Rachel's childlessness was that it led people to say that she wasn't worthy. Trying to set up a nation that's supposed to have God's endorsement when people are whispering that one of the founders seems not to be all that endorsed—it's a degrading situation. Thus, by choosing Joseph's name, Rachel praised God for saving her (and with her, the family mission) from humiliation.

A Final Point

When Rachel gives birth to Joseph, she does *not* say, "At last! I've finally succeeded in having my own child!"

Why not? That's what I would expect her to say. After all of her pain, shouldn't she feel that she finally got what she *really* wanted? But she doesn't express that at all. Astonishing.

It seems that after her argument with Jacob, and the further process of giving him her handmaid, Rachel *no longer felt that having a biological child was her primary goal.*

She realized that her lack of a biological child was definitely a legitimate personal problem. But it was *not* a loss to the mission that Jacob was involved in. She could be equally involved through her handmaiden's offspring.

This is monumental maturity and wisdom: to be able to differentiate between legitimate personal problems and world tragedies; to be able to assess my personal heartbreak—not as God's problem, not as a national emergency—as just something that I'm in terrible pain over.[7]

When Rachel finally did have a biological child, there was no sense of "at last," no hint of *"this* is what I really wanted the whole time." By the time she gave birth, it *wasn't* all she wanted anymore. She already *had* everything she wanted. The only negative element left had been her humiliation with regard to the family mission, which was removed with the birth of Joseph, her own biological child.

---

[1] Sforno again comments on the method: "That the *jealousy* of my friend should stimulate the nature." (Genesis 30:2)

[2] In case you're curious, I flipped back to find out who named Sarah's surrogate son. God, in a prophecy to Hagar, tells her to name her son Ishmael, from "God has heard your [Hagar's] pain/prayer." (Genesis 16:11.)

[3] Two letters of the Hebrew root are transposed: F"TL vs. T"FL. There are other similar cases of this reversal in the order of letters of a root.

[4] He comments on *niftalti*: My [Rachel's] prayer was accepted (Genesis 30:8).

[5] Rabbi Pelcovitz's interpretation, page 159.

[6] Just a friendly reminder: God doesn't forget/remember. That would imply change. It's just a way of expressing divine intervention.

[7] Tune in to Hannah's chapter for her argument that it *is* God's problem.

Chapter IX

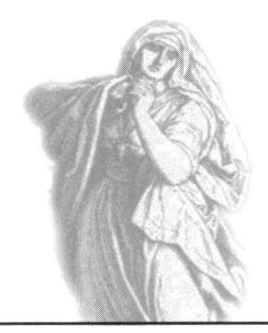

Leah and Rachel's Sibling Rivalry

Leah

Let's go back in time, before Joseph was born to Rachel, to see how Leah handled her period of infertility between the births of Reuven, Shimon, Levi, and Yehuda and the later births of Issachar, Zevulun, and Dina. (Remember, Rachel gave birth to her first-born son, Joseph, only after Leah had given birth to her last child, Dina.)

Secondary Infertility?

> And Leah saw that she had stopped giving birth; and she took Zilpah her maidservant and gave her to Jacob as a wife. And Zilpah the maidservant of Leah bore Jacob a son. And Leah said, "Good luck has come!" and she named him Gad. Zilpah the maidservant of Leah bore a second son to Jacob. Leah said, "In my good fortune! Because women have deemed me fortunate!" and she named him Asher [from the root *happy* or *fortunate*]. (Genesis 30:9-13.)

> God hearkened to Leah; and she conceived and bore Jacob a

fifth son. Leah said, "God has given me my reward because I gave my maidservant to my husband," and she named him Issachar [from the root to *reward*]. (Genesis 30:17-18.)

Deductions

Note that God "hearkened" to Leah, again implying that a Matriarch prayed.

When Leah stops conceiving, she uses Rachel's method, which was originally Sarah's method. What is her intention? Is she doing it so that she herself will conceive again? Or to increase her involvement in building the nation?

There is a bit of irony here. Trying to make yourself into a person with clear, true, principles only in order to get what you want will backfire. We've said that changing yourself[1] is the key to stimulating divine intervention. But going through the motions to get what you want won't help. Part of the process of self-improvement is letting go of certain expectations and claims—really, truly letting go.

We can see that in Leah's case. Both of the names of her sons from her maidservant express her great joy. *These* children are the source of her joy. Not because she's secretly hoping to have another child of her own later. She is genuinely happy to have greater participation in the development of the nation.

And yet, we see that, when she does conceive a child, Leah clearly considers Issachar to be a reward for giving her maidservant to her husband.

Rewards: Fact and Fiction

What is a reward? The classic concept of reward is based on the premise that the human being does not want to engage in a painful activity; if he performs the painful activity, he is rewarded. The reward heaps more pleasure on the scale when he is calculating the payoff: "pain vs. pleasure: is this worth doing?"

I tell Billy to brush his teeth. The reward is a dazzling smile, no fillings, and a full set of teeth when he's a senior citizen. But Billy doesn't care about that right now, and he hates brushing his teeth, so I pay him a quarter every time he does; I *reward* him for brushing his teeth.

If we try to fit this concept of reward into Leah's situation, we're going to get a little stuck.

Let's try it out. Here's Leah. The reward of giving her maidservant to her husband is: first, that the maidservant has children for Leah to participate in raising; second, that by creating an opportunity for jealousy to hold sway she will be sensitized to the reality of her situation.

Leah doesn't appreciate those benefits, so she gets a different reward: she gives birth to her own child.

That doesn't work at all. In fact, it contradicts our whole argument. It was only *because* she appreciated the benefit of giving her maidservant that she was rewarded with giving birth to her own child.

So what's a reward?

Apparently, thinking of a reward as something pleasurable to make up for something painful is a childish way of looking at it. Leah is telling us what a reward really is.

You start with a plan. You work hard to make the plan succeed. It does.

Is that a reward? When your plans work? That's not a reward, that's simply you doing what the world is designed to do (along with your own willingness to observe your emotional state and the good fortune of having all the factors you can't control work out).

A reward is when you get an extra, unanticipated result that is even more than the best result you were hoping for. Now *that's* a reward.

You put in all that effort because you have a goal. Here's an example. You spend three years watching your close friend, who had ignored a lump in her breast, fade away from chemotherapy. After seeing her suffer, you vow to raise awareness for breast cancer. Women should have regular mammograms; early detection means the difference between life and death—between surgery and dying from radiation poisoning and rampant cancer cells. You go on tours quoting statistics and urging women to make regular appointments.

What would you consider success? Every single woman who had been avoiding the test but now, because of your efforts, catches her cancer early enough to fight it, is your success.

A reward, on the other hand, is *more* than success. A reward is when, let's say, a doctor comes to hear you speak. She is so moved by your appeal that she decides to donate her time and a portable mammography machine, and accompany you on your circuit. Now women who are inspired by your appeal are able to get screened on the spot, before their motivation wears off.

Do you see what I mean? A reward is not something you can separate from the effort. It is not something that "makes up for" your pain.

It is also not a substitute for the benefit of your hard work. Your hard work based on a solid plan, that puts you in sync with the universe, will produce results. These results *are* the benefit.

A reward is in the same category as the benefit—it is the satisfaction of your efforts. The doctor with the portable mammogram unit helps to make your efforts successful in the same way, only more so, that your lectures themselves make your efforts successful.

Now I'll apply the same interpretation to Leah. Leah's goal was to help build the nation. Like Rachel, she was delighted with the sons of her maidservant. Her plan was a success. And then when she had a biological son, it satisfied her goal in a way that even *exceeded* her anticipated results—so she named him Issachar, "reward."

Interestingly, Leah got "rewarded" before Rachel. Gasp! I know what you're thinking. Does that mean that Leah was on a higher spiritual level than her sister? Not so fast. Remember what we learned from Sarah and Hagar? Results don't necessarily reveal a person's level of spirituality.

Are you dying to analyze Rachel and Leah's rivalry? I know I am.

Sibling Rivalry?

The thought of competition between Rachel and Leah appeals to the *yenta*, or busybody, in all of us. It's like a soap opera: two sisters, married to the same man, one having baby after baby while her barren sister looks on, the other passionately loved by the man while her more fertile sister is surrounded by babies whose names reflect her yearning for her husband's love.

It's easy to imagine that Rachel and Leah were involved in a competition for Jacob. One had his love, the other his children. Leah wanted to use her children to win Jacob's favor. Rachel had Jacob's love, and she wanted children.

To me, the biggest argument *against* this being a purely emotional competition is divine intervention. What kind of God involves Himself in a petty squabble between two people scuffling for superiority? "And Rachel said, 'Struggles of God have I struggled with my sister, and I too have succeeded.'" (Genesis 30:8.) If her words just mean that Rachel was trying to get the best of Leah, why would God help Rachel out? What makes her more deserving than Leah?

We've already discussed Sforno's noble explanation that Rachel and Leah were a team, struggling together to create a nation. Team effort aside, Sforno doesn't comment on the nuance of jealousy that flows through the story.

"And Rachel saw that she didn't bear children to Jacob, and Rachel was jealous of her sister." (Genesis 30:1.)

The question really is, why does Rachel name her son Naftali after her jealousy/struggle with her sister?

(What's in a Name? II) or A Rose by any Other Name

Why would Rachel want to give her son a name, Naftali, that would immortalize her struggle with her sister? Every time she calls her son, she will be reminded of the "struggles of God" she struggled with her sister.

"And I, too, have succeeded." (Genesis 30:8.) What did Rachel succeed at? Did she succeed in foiling her sister? Is she really expressing triumphant glee every time she calls her son?

That doesn't make sense. Even assuming the pettiest of motives (which we can't without getting stuck with a petty God who takes sides), that explanation doesn't hold water. *Leah* is the one who wants to foil her sister and win Jacob's love. *Rachel* just wants a child. When she succeeds, she's not gloating over Leah. Leah has four biological children to Rachel's two surrogate children. What's there to gloat about?

You might call it a triumph that Rachel has Jacob's love *and* two children, while Leah just has her children. I don't agree; if that were the case, Rachel would have named her *first* surrogate child for her triumph, once she had reached the status of having Jacob's love *and* his child. That would have been the ideal time to rejoice over her victory, if that's what she intended. The fact that she used her first child's name, Dan, to acknowledge God's justice leads me in a different direction.

Okay, back to square one. Why name a child after jealousy and struggle? What triumph is she talking about?

I think if we understand what Rachel considered to be a triumph, we'll understand why she wanted to keep the struggle in the forefront of her mind by naming her child after it.

Ibn Ezra is our most challenging commentator. I'll refresh our memory, since I'm sitting here with his commentary in front of me and you're probably not. On verse 8, on the word "struggles" he comments: "Its meaning is like a person who wrestles with another and struggles to beat him in order to topple him...The verse mentions God (*struggles of God have I struggled*) because it was for the honor of God that I gave my maidservant. Or God helped me in my wrestling."

What makes Ibn Ezra's commentary tricky is that at first glance he seems to be proving what I am so painstakingly trying to demonstrate is impossible; i.e. that Rachel and Leah are in a struggle of sibling rivalry.

I mean, come on, wrestling, trying to topple—doesn't it imply that Rachel is trying to "beat" Leah?

Take a closer look, though. Even in Ibn Ezra's own words we see that theory doesn't pan out, because he's trying to explain what God is doing in there.

It was for the honor of God that I gave my maidservant. That contradicts the theory of Rachel trying to one-up Leah. She did not give her maidservant to Jacob so that she could have both his love and his child, thus scoring higher than Leah. Ibn Ezra explicitly says that she did it for the honor of God. She wanted to participate in the mission started by Abraham and Sarah. She wanted to help produce a nation that rejects idolatry and lets the world know about the true Creator of the universe who runs everything.

Or God helped me in my wrestling. This also contradicts the idea that Rachel was trying to one-up Leah. As we said before, why praise a God who helps you one-up someone undeservedly?

Here's what I mean. Let's say somebody—a perfectly righteous somebody, just rather annoying—really gets on my nerves, so I hatch a plan to damage this annoying somebody. I'm successful, so I praise God. I would be praising God because He does what I want Him to do. That would imply a deity whose job is to run the universe according to my whims, but it would not be the true God of justice.

Okay, all that makes sense, but we still have Rachel trying to topple Leah.

Is Rachel's triumph referring to victory over Leah? Or is it something else?

The plain meaning of the verse is that Rachel has been victorious in her goal: to have a child. So what does that have to do with struggling with Leah? What is it about her struggle with Leah that led her to this victory of having a child?

Rachel's jealousy of her sister Leah caused her to embark on the process that ultimately led to her victory. As we said before, sometimes pain leads us to consider things about ourselves and about the world around us that we never would have given a second thought. Rachel's name "Naftali" commemorates the concept that the very great pain that causes introspection and reevaluation can ultimately lead to great joy.

---

[1] By growing into greater understanding, i.e. insight into the design of the universe, leading to enlightened action.

Chapter X

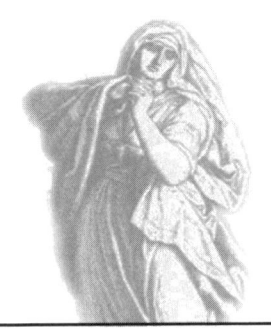

The Matriarchs' Stories: What Does It All Mean?

Why Did God Do This?

We've read what the Torah says about the Matriarchs. Since the wisdom of the Torah is infinite, we didn't finish. But now we have something to chew on. There are a few general questions that we asked earlier. I think we have enough background to look at them now. We asked:

Was there a purpose to the infertility of the Matriarchs?

If so, *what* was the purpose of their infertility?

Can that purpose apply to me if my infertility is not providentially determined, but rather a result of the laws of nature?

And of course, the questions that are really on our minds:

Why would God *do* this? And why is He doing this to *me*?

Serious questions. Let's see what we can do with them.

Let's start with the most pressing question. Why is God doing this to *me*?

As I mentioned earlier, this may be a divine decree, but then again it may not. God designed a system with laws of nature. To use a grossly anthropomorphic image, God can sit back, put his feet up, and let the world run according to the laws He designed.

We don't have a prophet to tell us whether our infertility stems from the laws of nature or whether God specifically decreed it in our cases. However, we do have knowledge of our own psychology. Human beings, when tragedy strikes, think, "Why *me*?"

I might think to reject the "Why *me*?" question on the grounds that I'm not even sure if I've been specially selected for infertility, but that would be hasty. God knows that this question looms in our minds; after all, He created us that way. The question "Why *me*?" is the gateway to discovery.

"Why *me*?" leads to another question: "Why am I infertile? Is there something awry in my relationship to children which would explain why God has punished me in this specific area?"[1]

Shock. Horror. Of course not! I love children! I want children!

Hold on. Slow down. A woman, even before she becomes a mother, has a relationship to her children. She has a mind-set, attitudes, and maternal feelings. She has an image of what being a mother will be like, what her children will be like, what her life as a mother with children will be like. You may be aware of these feelings or you may not.

If you have been frustrated in your attempt to have a child, now is the time to dig into these attitudes. It is time to explore. What attitudes might I have that can harm my child?

Try the following exercise. Write down, without self-censorship, the first thing that comes to your mind. Write as many answers as you can.

Why do you want to have a child?

_____
_____
_____
_____
_____
_____

Here is what I wrote, in the order in which I thought of them (which probably says something about their unconscious significance to me):

My List
Because they're so cute!
So I can feel like I've accomplished something.
So that a piece of me will live on after I'm gone.
So I can have something to love.
So that I can have something that will love me.
Because all of my friends have them.
Because people treat a pregnant woman like she's absorbed in the sacred privilege of carrying on the human race.
So I can feel like I'm worth something.
So I will be needed in a way that only a child needs his/her Mommy.
So people will admire my baby when I walk down the street.
It gives me a sense of purpose.
To make me feel fulfilled.
What greater accomplishment is there than to create a new life and help it turn into a person?
A responsibility to perpetuate the species (that was my husband's contribution).
To improve my marriage.
I really want to buy those adorable tiny clothes!
I'm bored.
I'm married; it's what I'm supposed to do.

That's my list. Did I miss any? Glancing over my reasons, some appear more ridiculous than others. It pays to catch the "silly" ones, though.

When I had my first miscarriage, the emotion that hit me the hardest (after "My baby is gone!" and "These kinds of things aren't supposed to happen to *me!*") was "Now I won't be pregnant at the same time as my sister and my close friend anymore!" That was, believe it or not, the main reason I was so depressed. But I didn't consciously know it because every time this thought came into my head I would think, "That's a ridiculous reason to be sad. There must be a more important reason you're so upset about this, like the loss of a potential life." But that didn't resonate. True, I was also upset for all of the "real" reasons, but those weren't causing the lurking sense of regret.

You might have a sense that wanting mini-accessories is not a "good" reason to want a baby. But why not?

And is it any different than "So that my life will have a sense of purpose"?

You Ain't Fit to Raise Kids

Ouch. I mean that in the most helpful way possible. Let me explain!

Month after month went by. Each month, for a few weeks, I was hopeful, expectant. Then disappointment hit like a punch in the stomach. Then stoicism set in. Then the cycle began again. Hope, expectation…

After a certain point I began making inquiries into my physical status. Am I ovulating? Is there anything else wrong with the plumbing?

As time continued to pass, I began to wonder if there was another approach to take in tandem with the physical investigation. If I'm looking into causes of my infertility, there is another possibility besides the physical. God designed the world so that the pain in any situation can help a person discover and reflect on the flaws in his character. In some cases, the pain is tailored to the individual, as an educational process to him to help him gain insight. "And know with your heart that the way a man chastises his son, the Lord, your God, chastises you." (Deuteronomy 8:5.) Was it possible that if I looked at the pain I was in, and saw how it was related to character flaws, that my infertility would stop?

It was a very primal thought process. "Me in pain. Me want to be out of pain. If uncovering distortions and misunderstandings in this area will get me out of pain, Me on board."

When a woman is infertile, she naturally asks, "Why me? Is this a divine punishment?" The next question is, "If it is a punishment, why is it not being able to have children? Is God trying to tell me that I don't deserve to have children? Why don't I deserve to have children?"

Remember: this does *not* mean that infertile women do not deserve to have children. Those are just the natural thoughts that go through an infertile woman's head. Since those thoughts are there, this is the method I used to capitalize on them. I hoped that this method would help me, the infertile woman, identify where my goals and God's goals contradict each other. God is not inclined to intervene on behalf of people whose goals contradict His goals (as you recall from our discussion of divine intervention).[2]

This was the method I used. I describe it to you here in the hopes that it can be useful to you as well. I began, as systematically as I could, to try to discover why I wanted children. I had many opportunities to think about it—every time I saw a woman with her baby on the street, every time I heard someone was pregnant, every time a fresh wave of pain washed over me, I tried to understand my reactions. Why does it hurt? What do I feel?

The months passed—still no pregnancy. I looked further and deeper into my hopes and dreams for a child. What I saw gave me pause. Any or all of my reasons for wanting a child could actually interfere with raising a well-adjusted, healthy child.

A strong statement; I know. How can having a child so that I can have something to love be a bad thing? Everyone knows children need love.

Any reason that you have for wanting a child has the potential to blind you into making mistakes when you raise that child. Sounds crazy, right?

It all comes down to what we think children are for. I began to realize, sifting through my feelings, that all of my different, complicated, multi-textured feelings about my future child had a definite common theme.

Is the child something to make me feel certain things about myself, or is the child its own person? A separate, alive-in-its-own-right being that ultimately has nothing to do with me and has the right to go off and exist on its own? (A friend of mine once said, when questions are phrased like that, the answer is usually "b")

Sure, no problem. Something to make me feel good, or his or her own person? Let's see. The second one, definitely "his or her own person." (Told you it was "b") Great. But—

When I was thinking of my future child, I was always thinking of it in terms of myself. How much *I* wanted it. How *I* would feel about it. What *I* would do with it. How it would make *me* feel. Even "I want to do something that has a real purpose" can be phrased as "I will feel good doing something that has a real purpose," i.e., I'm doing it because of how it will make *me* feel.

This is all fine and dandy; after all, at this point, there *was* no baby. There was only me. If I'm embarking on an activity, I'm going to do it because of how *I* feel about it.

But as I thought about it, I began to think that the very reasons that motivated me to want children might backfire when I was confronted with an actual live child.

Having children is like giving gifts. Who is the gift for, the giver or the receiver? We might assume it's the recipient. But have you ever opened a jewelry box only to find a gaudy bauble resting on the elegant velvet, and the giver's hopeful eyes and expectant smile have you saying, "Oooooh! It's perfect!"? Giver or receiver? The giver puts so much thought into it, wants to get a certain reaction, has expectations about your gratitude...

When you're a parent, it's like you're giving your child a gift, the gift of his own existence. Logically, that gift now belongs to him (or her).[3] But I have expectations, hopes, dreams about how I want that child to turn out, how I want that child to interact with me, and how I want that child to be around others as a reflection of me, my efforts and values.

I started noticing all of the different ways that I wanted to use my future child to make me feel good about myself:

"Oh, look at that mother walking her baby. I want to be walking down the street and have people see me, the picture of satisfied maternity."

"Look at that toddler nuzzle her Mommy's neck. I want someone to feel that way about me."

"Look at that tiny little hand. I want to marvel at my own baby's tiny hand and be amazed that I gave birth to this creature."

"Look at those mothers talking about their children's schools. I want to participate."

My stomach clenched every time I saw a joy that I was missing. After a while, I started to see: Each joy I imagined was based on a *value* that I held dear.

Do you know what I mean? Feelings don't come from nowhere; they're the result of my values.

Let's go back to that poignant image of me, a mother, feeling joy that I gave birth to this tiny, complete creature. Feel my amazement and bliss.

That joy is because I value thinking of myself as "Me, Giver of Life."

"Have a party, Jess. Enjoy the pleasure," I told myself. "But what happens when this darling baby doesn't seem to appreciate you as the grand caregiver? When your toddler looks you straight in the eye and throws her bowl of spaghetti and tomato sauce on the floor? Or when your teenager curses you, stomps upstairs to his room and slams the door?"

Will I be so attached to this vision of myself that I'll get annoyed at my child for trampling all over it? Or will I be able to parent him firmly and appropriately, without being blinded by the threat it poses to my self-image?

You may not relate to those example; they are specific to my personal character flaws. Let's try another.

The Joy of the Contented Mother Shepherding her Adorable, Loving Children

What is the value that causes this particular happiness? There are lots of values. Hmm...having well-behaved children, having children who treat me and themselves with respect, being perceived by other people as a good mother, feeling like motherhood is something I'm good at, feeling like my children are something I can be proud of...

Now, if Sibling #3 (we should be so lucky as to have multiple children) is acting out his sibling rivalry by ruthlessly tormenting Sibling #2 (who keeps wailing "Mommmmmmy! Make him stop!") while Sibling #1 is anxious that her best friend at school won't like her unless she's cool, and therefore whines non-stop that she needs a $150-pair of shoes in order to be popular, how will I handle it?

Am I able to see clearly why these children are behaving the way they are and respond with an approach that supports their best interests? Or do I just get angry at them because they're threatening my values?

And what would I teach them if I hissed "Shut up, kids, you're embarrassing me!" instead of parenting them through their individual issues? ("Number three and number two, you're separated. You stand on my left and you on my right. Number one, it sounds like you want those shoes very badly.") Instead of setting safe, reassuring limits and helping them gain control when they're overwhelmed, I would be teaching them that their lack of control threatens my image of myself and causes me to lose control, too.

Back to the Matriarchs

Infertility can inspire a person to examine his or her desire for children. It is ideal, when building a nation, to be aware of the personal gratification that you're seeking through your children.[4] The Matriarchs were able to shape their children's lives based on their understanding of the design of God's universe. Instead of being distracted by a vision of how they wanted their children to turn out, they were able to see their *actual* children. They thus created a nation of people whose goal is to reflect the existence of a Creator.

They Ain't Fit Either; How Come They Get To?

It's not fair! Why do I have to perfect my motivations when the whole world (aside from the millions of other infertile people per year) is having babies without going through this process?

I always thought it smacked of a cosmic joke that God designed human beings' prime child-bearing years as ages fourteen through thirty, when people have youth without the knowledge that comes with experience. By the time you have collected enough wisdom to know what you're doing, you're too old to have kids (and your kids want to make their own mistakes with your grandkids; they are unlikely to want to listen to your advice). What started off as an amusing observation became a bitter pill as I struggled to gain insight into my motivations for having children. There I was, standing on the sidelines, as people casually and unthinkingly parented their way through their progeny.

That question bothered me as I went through this process. To some extent, it still bothers me. I see that I'm better off after this process. In fact, I still shudder a bit when I think about me raising children without the discoveries I've made about what I'm trying to get from my children. And I also shudder a bit when I stop to imagine how much I didn't uncover. There's a part of me that's sorry I stopped thinking about it as soon as I got pregnant, even though I'm mostly relieved not to be thinking about it anymore. There's only so much a person can take about her unconscious motivations. Once I no longer had the pain to motivate me, I gratefully fled from introspection. Despite all the wonderful benefits of infertility (read that tongue-in-cheek), I resent that I had to go through so much pain of honest evaluation, while so many women blithely pop 'em out one after the other, never needing to take a moment to question if their attitudes towards their children are possibly damaging those children.

Here's how I understand the answer to the "It's Not Fair" question, as best as I can see it.

What's really bothering me? Not the awareness that my personal emotions could negatively affect my children; that's a good thing. Nope, it's the process that kills me. How come *I* had to go through so much pain? Why doesn't *everybody* have to go through this pain? I wouldn't mind going through it if it were par for the course. "Everybody who wants to have children, sign on the dotted line here, go stand in line there, and wait for your pain. You will go through X months of introspection and soul-searching until you have gained some insight into the possible mistakes you would make. Following this process, you can have your baby. Here you go."

That's what I think it comes down to. It bothers me that I've been singled out[5] for pain. I don't think that I should have to go through more pain than other people. When it comes down to it, there's a part of me that would love to be ignorantly parenting and harming my kids, rather than have to be one of the not-so-many people who have to agonize about what's really motivating them.

Wow. Let's go over that again. There's a part of me that might negatively affect my own children, rather than force me to confront my own distorted opinions. I'm going to sit here and ponder that for a while. You go on ahead.

What If I Never Have Children?

What happens if I never have children? What is the point of knowing the reality of the purpose of having children? What happens if I uncover every angle of how I might try to gratify myself with my child at the expense of my child—and then never have a child? How does this help me? Does this help me?

As a person who now has children, maybe I have no business asking this question. Maybe it's your own private and personal anguish. But it's incomplete to talk about the necessity to go through this process if I don't address the very real possibility that you may still be childless at the end of it.

I actually do not feel qualified to discuss it. I can see certain things, but I'm afraid of sounding like that callous pamphlet I told you about that I received with my IUI packet. The one that suggested I explore the option of child-free living. Coldhearted jerks. I may say it in such a way that you slam this book closed, hurl it across the room, and chase it down to stomp all over it.

And you'd be justified. Who am I to give you insight about childlessness? I don't know what I'm talking about. I don't know how it *feels* to be told "give up." It's hopeless. There's no chance. That the only possibility is one of those "miracle babies" that you periodically hear about. (My aunt's husband's sister actually had one of those. The doctors said she would never conceive, but she did.) There are only two choices: you can continue to have your hopes invested in an infinitesimal possibility, or you can try to move on. Adjust to your "child-free" situation. Or find a needy parentless child who will thrive with your love.

For what it's worth, I'll share what I've been able to understand. Don't feel bad if you cry all over the page or throw this at the wall.

Sarah and Rachel are the role models in this discussion. Sarah did not expect to have children, and Rachel went through a lengthy process to become satisfied with her situation, even though she couldn't have children.

Rachel is particularly inspiring to me, because she ultimately considered her inability to have children as a personal problem, instead of a cosmic problem.

Every time I think about this issue, the following example keeps coming into my head (Disclaimer: believe me, I am well aware that having children is a far deeper emotional issue than the desire expressed in this example.)

I once heard someone say, "I really, really want to go to Hawaii. If I died and never made it to Hawaii, I think that I'd be missing something from my life. I will be really upset if I end up not making it to Hawaii."

With all due respect to the beauty of Hawaii (I've never been there), I remember thinking, "Are you serious? Are you really seriously suggesting that your life will be missing an essential element of meaning without Hawaii?"

Hawaii may be beautiful. In fact, it may be *the most* beautiful, fun, wonderful place in the whole world. But to posit that your life will be lacking if you miss out on this experience…you're missing the whole point.

Life is not defined by the enjoyable experiences of your life. Life is defined by *You*. What kind of person were you? What kind of insights did you have? How did your insights express themselves in action?

It seems that Rachel got to the point where having her own child was like visiting Hawaii. She thought it would be a wonderful, pleasurable experience, one that she wanted desperately. She realized that ultimately, if she went through life and never merited this experience, she would be in pain. But she had a certain perspective that it would be nothing more than the pain of a missed experience. It would not take away from who she is as a person, and it would not compromise the value of her life.

It would, however, be an experience that she would continuously, sorrowfully miss.

Beyond the Matriarchs: It's Not Personal and it is Personal

You may have noticed that there are a lot of pages still to go in this book. Indeed, we have looked at all four of the Matriarchs from Genesis, but the Bible contains many more books of wisdom for the harvesting.

Let's get our feet wet (to mix agricultural and aquatic metaphors) with some fascinating passages.

It's Not Personal

In Exodus 23:25-26, God describes a state of society where there is no infertility:

> And serve the Lord your God and He will bless your bread and your water, and remove illness from your midst. There will be no woman who loses her young [*i.e., through miscarriage or stillbirth*—Rashi] or is infertile in your land; I will fill the number of your days.[6]

Also in Deuteronomy 7:12-14:

> And it will be, if you listen to these laws and guard them and do them, then the Lord your God will guard the covenant and kindness that he swore to your forefathers. And he will love you and bless you and multiply you, and he will bless the fruit of your womb and the fruit of your land, your grain, your wine, and your oil, the offspring of your cattle and the flocks of your sheep and goats on the land that He swore to your forefathers to give you. You will be the most blessed of all the peoples; there won't be an infertile male or infertile female among you nor among your animals.

What's going on here? Is God making a trade?[7] You serve me, and I'll reward you with no illness, famine or infertility?

What are we supposed to understand from this? Do we deduce that any infertility or illness in our society is a signal that we're not serving God correctly? That's hard to believe. Illness strikes us because we're sinners?

No! In fact, these verses are telling us the *opposite*.

I know, God told us in Exodus about a state of society with no illness or infertility. A state directly related to our service of God. But we have to look at that idea carefully.

These verses are telling us something we don't really like to hear. (Intrigued yet?)

Because physical matter (the stuff the whole universe is made of) is so adaptable, it leads to all sorts of structural weaknesses and defects. Let's take a look at wood as an example. Wood is so great to work with because you can chop it, sand it, and shape it to take on whatever form you want. Wood is very versatile, which is why we love using it so much. But—that's also why it breaks and gets worn. The problem is, once it's the shape you want (a table with a smooth surface) you don't want it to change shape anymore (get covered with nicks when your neighbor's little darling drums on your table with the car keys). But that's the nature of wood. It can't stop being wood-like, and thus, easy to form, once it's the shape *you* want it to be. It's susceptible to wear and tear.

It's like that with everything. Sickness and infertility happen because people are made of cells and organs and the very adaptability of those things also means they're disposed to breaking. There are all sorts of bacteria floating around that help our ecosystem and keep the cycle of life going, but that means that our cells sometimes get attacked. You can't say, "Well, I like rain, but I don't like flooding." Flooding sometimes happens because rain is rain and does what rain does. You can't say, "Well, I wish that cells had the ability to grow and repair themselves, but not to make fibroids." You don't have to like them, but if you waved your magic wand and removed the cause of fibroids, you'd also be removing something you do benefit from. The two are not separable.

Rav Hirsch says that these two passages are talking about "the natural illnesses and weaknesses which, under the regime of Nature, are considered indispensable from Human life."[8] These things happen because nature is the way it is; most of the time, this works out great, but some of the time it leads to illness.

So if you should be a victim of these "natural weaknesses and illnesses," it is not necessarily an indication of your personal state. It's a statement that society does not merit "hyper-Providence," protection even from normal illnesses.

It is Personal

Lest you be heaving a sigh of relief that God is not out to get *you*, don't relax yet. It's not that simple. (Well, as far as God being "out to get" anybody, it *is* that simple. If you're imagining "out to get," then you're imagining a scenario where God is being gratified by putting you through pain. God does not get emotional satisfaction from putting people in pain.)

The question "Is my infertility a punishment for a specific sin that I committed, or is it a result of the laws of nature?" is only answerable via a prophet, and the likelihood that you will encounter one to give you an answer is very slim, as we noted earlier. So we have to puzzle this through on our own.

We've just looked at some sources that show us that infertility can be nothing personal, just a result of the laws of nature. Now let's take a look at the other possibility.

---

[1] Thanks, Marshall Gisser, for directing me to this question.

[2] When I say God has "goals," I'm not making any statement about His motivation, rather than in the same way you can see that a chair is designed for sitting, if you study a design you can see what it's for. Study a child. What is its design? Is that how I was thinking of a child?

[3] Let's agree that "him" means "him or her" and "he" means "he or she" and vice versa.

[4] Actually, this applies any time you're raising any child. But in the case of the Matriarchs, self-awareness (or lack of it) had national repercussions, even repercussions for all of humanity.

[5] Me, and millions of others.

[6] There are different opinions as to what exactly the phrase "fill the number of your days" means. It is generally understood to mean that people will die of old age.

[7] Be careful! It can't be the kind of trade where God is in a weak position, desperately bargaining so that He can get something that He needs (i.e. our service).

[8] Hirsch, *Pentateuch Translation and Commentary: Deuteronomy*, page 416.

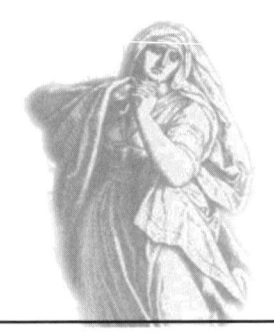

Chapter XI

Michal

Samuel II 6:15-16; 20-23:

And David and the entire house of Israel brought up the ark of God with loud, joyous sound and the sound of the *shofar*. And it was that the ark of God came to the City of David, and Michal [King David's wife] the daughter of Saul peered out the window and saw King David leaping and joyously dancing before God and she degraded him in her heart...And David returned to bless his household, and Michal the daughter of Saul came out to greet David and she said, "How honored today was the King of Israel, who was exposed to the eyes of his servant's maidservants, the way an empty-headed person would be exposed!" And David said to Michal, "Before God, who chose me over your father[1] and his whole household to appoint me as leader of the nation of God on Israel—I will rejoice before God. And I would have degraded myself even more, and been low in my eyes, and among the maidservants that you spoke of—among them I would be honored! [i.e., people do consider it honorable to behave this way for the honor of God]." And Michal the daughter of Saul didn't have a child until the day she died.

The commentators are unanimous: Michal was punished with infertility for what she said to King David. There are different opinions as to whether she had children before this incident took place, and whether she died in childbirth ("didn't have a child until the day she died" is an ambiguous phrase). There are also different opinions about whether Michal spoke to David privately, or criticized him publicly. ("And Michal the daughter of Saul came out to greet David and she said...")

Divine punishment is educational. The pain caused by the punishment is like a red flag urgently demanding, "Look over here! Here's a character flaw!"

What was Michal's mistake? Why was the punishment infertility? What is the connection between infertility and Michal's criticism of King David?

King David and Michal seem to be arguing about the concept of a king's dignity: should the king maintain his dignity when expressing joy before God? King David explains that the king doesn't deserve honor for his own sake; the people respect the king as an agent of God's will, the leader of a society that represents the existence of God to all of humanity. Dancing wildly to celebrate the return of the ark brings honor to God's name.

This particular interchange doesn't do justice to King David and Michal's relationship. The Talmud (Sanhedrin 21a) describes how beloved Michal was to King David. Check out Samuel I 15:11-17 to read about how Michal audaciously saved David's life when her own father was trying to kill him.[2]

It's hard to figure out exactly what Michal did to warrant the punishment of infertility. In fact, some commentators[3] link Michal's mistake back to an error her father, King Saul, had made—an error that cost his line the dynasty. (Take a look at Samuel I 15 if you want to try to see what exactly King Saul did wrong.) Michal's error was similar to the one that cost King Saul the kingdom; evidently, she did not merit progeny who would be part of the dynasty, either.

I don't bring this up to analyze Michal's personal story. I think there is a larger message for us here, beyond understanding her particular mistake. More globally, we see that infertility can be a divine decree, a punishment for a specific philosophical error that caused you to make a mistake (i.e., a "sin").

That's a possibility for any of us, and it pays to take it seriously. Happily, the constructive response to infertility is the same whether the infertility stems from divine punishment or whether it's the result of the laws of nature: look for a character flaw in yourself related to having children, understand what mistake you're making, and hope that your new insight will lead to divine intervention now that you are no longer blinded by goals that contradict God's plan.

It's finally time to take a look at prayer. We ask and God grants. Or is it that simple? A frail human who hardly controls his own existence has access to the Creator and can overturn nature's decrees. But how? Prayer is a powerful tool. And like any tool, knowing how to use it will help you get the results you want.

---

[1] Saul, Michal's father, was King of Israel before David, and lost the dynasty because he made a serious error (Samuel I 15).

[2] Talk about in-laws! Seriously, though, King Saul was a victim of mental illness towards the end of his life. In his moments of clarity, he spoke of David with the highest respect. David, in turn, always treated King Saul as a respected monarch.

[3] Malbim on Samuel II 6:23.

Chapter XII

Hannah

Rosh Hashana. The High Holy Days. The Days of Awe.

The Torah portion read in the synagogue on the first day of Rosh Hashana is Genesis 21, the story of Sarah—"And God remembered Sarah, as He had said; and God did for Sarah as He had spoken. And Sarah conceived, and gave birth..." The portion read from the Prophets is the story of Hannah (*Chana* in Hebrew). Two stories of women "remembered" by God.

God doesn't forget anything. "Remembering" is a term for divine intervention.

As I read the story of Hannah, I thought to myself, "It looks like this story unlocks some of the mysteries of how to bring about divine intervention. I should take a closer look at this story!" (Well, my words were more like: "Hey! She prayed and got a child. How did she do that? How do *I* do that?")

Let's take a closer look at this story.

Samuel I 1:1-23:

> There was one man from Ramasayim-Tzofim, from Mount Efraim, whose name was Elkana, son of Yerocham, son of Elihu, son of Tochu, son of Tzuf, from Efrat. And he had two wives: one's name was Hannah, and the second's name was Penina; and Penina had children and Hannah had no children. And this man would go up from his city from year to

year to prostrate himself and bring offerings to God, Master of Legions, in Shiloh [where the Tabernacle was. This was before the Temple was built], where the two sons of Eli, Chofni and Pinchas, were priests to God.

It happened on the day that Elkana brought offerings that he gave portions to Penina his wife and all of her sons and daughters. And to Hannah he gave a double portion, because he loved Hannah and God had closed her womb. Her adversary [i.e., co-wife] angered her again and again in order to cause her pain, because God had closed her womb.

This is what he would do year after year; when she would go up to the house of God, thus she would anger her, and she would cry and not eat. And Elkana her husband said to her, "Hannah, why do you cry and why do you not eat? And why is your heart broken? Aren't I better to you than ten sons?" [*Banim* can be translated as *sons* or *children*.]

And Hannah got up after she ate in Shiloh and after she drank; and Eli the priest was sitting on the chair next to the doorpost of the sanctuary of God. And she was bitter of spirit, and she prayed on God, and she cried greatly. And she made a vow and she said, "God, Master of Legions, if You take note of the suffering of Your maidservant, and remember me, and don't forget Your maidservant, and give to Your maidservant male offspring, then I will give him to God all the days of his life, and a razor will not come onto his head."

And it was as she increased praying before God that Eli was keeping an eye on her lips. And Hannah was speaking to her heart, just her lips were moving and her voice wasn't heard;

and Eli thought she was drunk. And Eli said to her, "How long will you be drunk? Remove your wine from yourself!" And Hannah answered, and she said, "No, my lord, I am a woman of aggrieved spirit, and wine and strong drink I haven't drunk, and I poured my soul before God. Don't consider your maidservant to be a base woman, because it is out of my grievance and anger I have been speaking [i.e., praying]." And Eli answered and said, "Go in peace, and may the God of Israel grant your request that you have asked of Him." And she said, "May your maidservant find favor in your eyes."

And the woman went on her way, and she ate, and she no longer had her upset face. They woke up in the morning and bowed before God, and returned and came to their house, to Ramah. And Elkana knew his wife Hannah, and God remembered her. And it was as the days passed, Hannah got pregnant and gave birth to a son, and she named him Samuel [*Shmuel* in Hebrew] because she requested [*sha'al*] him from God.

We see from verse 5 that Hannah was infertile ("and God had closed her womb"). We don't know how long this had already been going on, except that the story describes that "year after year" Elkana gave her a double portion to comfort her, and Penina provoked her.

This story is particularly exciting because we get a taste of the content of Hannah's prayer. What are the factors that caused Hannah's prayer to be answered?

Before we begin mining the story for insights into prayer, let's take a look at some points that struck me about Elkana and Penina.

You Don't Understand!

Is infertility harder on the husband or the wife?

That's a hard question to answer. Since men are less prone to sharing their feelings, women often assume that they don't feel as strongly. Infertility is painful in many different ways; in some areas, women take it harder, and in some ways, it's harder on men.

Women are usually hardest hit in two areas: the social arena and the thwarted maternal instinct. Women are the primary caregivers from many points of view: biologically, psychologically, and socially. When everyone around us has babies and everyone expects us to have babies, it creates unrelenting social torture. If that was not bad enough, I found myself battling my own urge for a baby the way a smoker trying to quit has to battle the craving for a cigarette. I never realized just how strong my maternal instinct was until it was frustrated. I just wanted to cuddle and care for a young life.

Men, as I understand it, learn to have tender feelings toward babies particularly after they have acquired one of their own.[1] They are born with nary a nurturing bone in their bodies. (I'm blithely generalizing here. I know it may not apply to you.) Men don't seem to be subject to the same urge for babies as women. Have you ever seen a group of men clustered around a newborn, cooing and begging to hold it while the glowing father cradles it protectively?

Interestingly, though, my husband was the one who pushed for me to enter treatment. I was conflicted. I thought maybe I should wait another six months to a year; since I was diagnosed with "unexplained infertility," I believed that there was a good chance that time was on my side.

I also think that men have a harder time with adoption than women (again, this does not apply to everyone). The great fulfillment of loving and nurturing a child seems to play a stronger role in satisfying maternal yearnings, rather than paternal drives. For men, a major component of their satisfaction in building a family is, well, the *building* part, the immortality aspect—conquering the world by populating it.

Infertility is like an ugly outfit—some people find the style offensive, some people can't take the color, some people shudder at the fabric, but nobody finds it attractive. Men and women alike have to cope with many painful aspects of infertility.

The aspects that bother the husband may bother the wife less and vice versa, which causes a common phenomenon—the perception on the part of the wife that her husband "doesn't understand" what she is going through. When the wife comes home sobbing, cut to the quick by a friend's careless comment, the husband can't relate. "What's the big deal?" he says, meaning to sound comforting as he pats his wife's heaving back. (A word to the wise: "What's the big deal?" is not a good thing to say to a crying woman.)

In fact, one of the most difficult things that men have to cope with during infertility is their wives' bewildering and intense pain, sometimes to the exclusion of coping with or discussing their own. I recently asked my husband, "Who do you think has a harder time with infertility, the man or the woman?" and he answered, without hesitation, "the woman." I asked him, "If that's the case, why were you the one who was so gung-ho for treatment while I was so hesitant?" He paused, considered, and then said, "I don't know."

Imagine that. During all the years we were coping with infertility, we never once had a conversation about my husband's pain. Maybe a sentence here and there, but he never fully articulated his feelings. As I recall, our conversations were mostly about both of us trying to cope with *my* feelings.

The story of Hannah reflects these different coping patterns. Elkana shows touching love and concern for his wife, but he seems puzzled about the depth of her pain. Let's look at it again:

> And to Hannah he gave a double portion, because he loved Hannah and God had closed her womb. Her adversary [i.e., co-wife] angered her again and again in order to cause her pain, because God had closed her womb. This is what he would do year after year; when she would go up to the house

of God, thus she would anger her, and she would cry and not eat. And Elkana her husband said to her, "Hannah, why do you cry and why do you not eat? And why is your heart broken? Aren't I better to you than ten sons?" And Hannah got up after she ate in Shiloh and after the drinking... (Samuel I 1:5-9.)

Elkana asks Hannah, "Aren't I better to you than ten sons?" What kind of a question is that? Why would a man think that having a good husband would be perceived as sufficient blessing by a woman despairing about her childlessness? They are two separate issues. There is having a good husband, which is certainly nothing to sneeze at, but is not the same as having children. You don't give birth to a husband. Your husband doesn't need you to survive—nor would you want him to. In the two main areas that an infertile woman feels bereft—in social belonging and satisfaction of maternal yearnings—a husband is not an adequate stand-in. You'd be better off with a puppy.

Well, now that I've bashed poor Elkana (and any of you husbands who may have dared to try a similar approach), let's try to understand what Elkana meant. He certainly was trying to comfort his beloved wife.

Hannah's Response

First let's note what Hannah *didn't* do. She didn't bite his head off and she didn't snap at him. It appears that she took his question as he had intended it—she understood that he wanted to comfort her. In fact, the commentators note that she did eat[2] though the text had just previously described that her grief was so great that she cried and didn't eat. Apparently, Elkana's urging comforted her enough to eat a little something.

Elkana's Attempt to Comfort Hannah

The Malbim, a nineteenth-century Eastern European commentator, notes that verse 8 tells us three things Elkana noticed about Hannah:

she was crying, she wasn't eating, and she was angry. What solution did he suggest? "But aren't I better to you than ten sons?" Malbim expands: "The woman isn't commanded to have children [in Judaism this commandment applies only to men, as we have discussed], and if you are concerned with having a staff for your hand and somebody to bury you, I will be there to help and protect you."

Every time I read this I'm struck by how...how *masculine* that answer is—how pragmatic. "Don't worry. If you're concerned about your relationship with God, your infertility doesn't pose an obstacle; it is not your obligation to have children. And if you're in pain because you won't have children to support you and help you, I can fill that role for you."[3]

It may seem like Elkana is giving a very practical answer, that doesn't really address her grief. Is the real emotional pain of barrenness that you will have no children to take care of you? Doesn't it involve so much more?

Maybe I'm not the only wife who does this, but I have a tendency to shrug off my husband's pragmatic solutions when I'm upset. I'm insulted that he's not "validating" my pain, as though he just wants me to stop hurting so he can go back to his football game with a clear conscience.

But maybe I'm being too hard on him. Maybe, like Elkana, he's just trying to be helpful in the areas where something can be done. Hannah is barren; she can't have children. Elkana accepts that. But he is trying to comfort her by shifting the focus to an arena where he does have some control. When it comes to satisfying her maternal yearnings, he's helpless; if the issue is relieving her social isolation, he can't. But in terms of the insecurity of having no one to take care of her, which is a practical problem—he can spare her that, and he will. It's a loving and generous offer, intended to comfort her in the only way he can.

Elkana inspires me to strive to be more gentle and understanding with my own husband when he offers a well-intentioned practical solution, even if it doesn't address my emotional pain.

Beyond the Practical to the Emotional

We understand now that Elkana, being male, is trying to console Hannah by offering comfort only in those areas where he has some influence. Doesn't that sound logical? "But honey, how can I comfort you for something that I can't do anything about? 'Empathy?' How would that help? It wouldn't fix anything!"

Two additional interpretations of Elkana's attempt to comfort Hannah follow the same train of thought. Both Rashi and Metzudas Dovid understand "Am I not as good to you as ten sons?" not to mean that Hannah should consider Elkana better than ten sons, but that Elkana considers *Hannah* better than ten sons. "I am as good to you as" means "my love for you is as valuable as" ten sons.

They disagree as to whose ten sons Elkana has in mind. Rashi says: "I love you more than the ten sons that Penina bore me." According to Rashi, Elkana is trying to comfort Hannah in the only way he can. He can't fix her infertility, but in case any aspect of Hannah's pain is due to her desire to give him children, he assures her that he is happy to be married to her and the emotional satisfaction of being married to her is more than the satisfaction he has from his existing children.

Metzudas Dovid says: "My desire for you is more than if you had borne ten sons." This line of reasoning is similar to Rashi's. If Hannah is concerned that Elkana might be dissatisfied with her because of her barrenness, he assures her that he loves her for herself, and that he would not love her any more if she had children.

Elkana cannot cure Hannah's barrenness, but he is anxious to put her mind at ease over any aspects of her pain that stem from concern for her husband and his opinion of her.

After she has something to eat, Hannah pours her heart out to

God. She is still in anguish—an anguish triggered by Penina's deliberate attempts to rile her up.

Penina

From her loving husband to her vicious co-wife, the characters surrounding Hannah weave a tapestry that unfurls into her prayer. What is so important about Hannah's torment? Why does the story comment on it?

> And her adversary would anger her; she would also anger her in order to enrage her, because God had closed her womb. And she would do this year after year whenever they would go up to the house of God; she would anger her in this way, and she would cry and not eat. (Samuel I 1:6-7.)

No One Can Make You Feel Inferior Without Your Consent[4]

Taken at face value, is Penina a malicious woman? According to Metzudas Dovid, she verbally tormented Hannah, angering her repeatedly (verse 6 says *"in order* to enrage her"). It seems that Penina was deliberately trying to infuriate Hannah.

What I am about to say is not intended to defend Penina in any way, though we will look at an alternative explanation for her behavior later. Penina faced severe consequences for the way she treated Hannah, as we'll soon see. But Metzudas Dovid makes an interesting comment; he quotes Chazal's claim that Penina used to joke around with Hannah, saying, "Oh, haven't you bought overalls for your oldest yet, or an undershirt for your youngest?" And he comments: "And there was room for Penina to anger her, because God had closed her womb...And she was bitter of spirit because of her infertility, and it was an easy matter to anger her."

That kind of joke doesn't have to be a deliberate vicious attack. But even if we think of it as unconscious aggression in the guise of rueful sympathy, it still stings. So what is Metzudas Dovid getting at? Penina was being mean. Hannah reacted. What does he mean by claiming that Hannah gave Penina room to anger her because she was easily angered?

Metzudas Dovid seems to be offering a valuable (if slightly painful) insight: there are two parties to every interaction. If I'm constantly feeling hurt, it pays to look at *my* contribution to the interactions. If I wear my belt up around my neck, then any time someone hits me I can accuse him of hitting below the belt. Part of the reason Hannah took Penina's teasing so hard is that the barbs were in an area where Hannah was predisposed to be sensitive.

How does that help? Penina is still the aggressive party here. And what can Hannah (or any of us) do if it turns out that we're *particularly* sensitive? So it turns out that I'm giving people room to hurt me because I'm sensitive. Does that make it my fault? And can I stop being sensitive? I can't turn off my feelings.

True. But just knowing that my sensitivity is a factor puts the situation in a different light. I've gone from "me, helpless victim," to "me, participant and contributor." Certainly not the primary contributor, and certainly not the aggressive contributor, but I can't totally blame the other person anymore. Since I'm a partner to the interaction, I can take more control. I can, for example, sheepishly confess that I am particularly sensitive about this topic and request a change of subject. And even if I don't speak up, even if I never say anything, I will still know that part of what causes me pain is my particular sensitivity.

The Consequences

Interestingly enough, it was Penina's behavior that ultimately caused Hannah to conceive. "And she was bitter of spirit and she prayed to God and she cried greatly." (Verse 10.) The intense pain motivated the prayer, the prayer led to divine intervention, and Hannah conceived.

The text hints, though it does not directly state, that Penina was severely punished for her teasing. When Hannah donates Samuel to the House of God, as she had vowed in her prayer that she would do, she prays again, this time a song of praise and thanks.

> My heart is happy with God, my horn is raised with God [to gore my enemies; i.e., I can finally defend myself against my tormentor Penina][5], my mouth is opened to my enemies because I am happy at Your salvation...The bow of the mighty breaks, and those who stumble gird with strength [suddenly fortunes can change according to the will of God]. Those who are satiated with bread have to rent themselves out as workers, and those who are starving can stop working, until a barren woman can give birth to seven children and one who has many children becomes bereft. (Samuel I 2:1,4-5.)

The basic reading of the text interprets mention of the barren woman and the mother of many as an illustration of how fortunes can suddenly change. Things in life may seem to be going well, but security is an illusion.

However, some of the commentators think that Hannah chose that particular example because it originated close to home—that it was a description of Hannah and Penina's own situation.[6]

Rashi expands, quoting Chazal: "When Hannah gave birth to one, Penina buried two—and she had ten children. When Hannah had given birth to four, Penina had buried eight, and when Hannah got pregnant and had her fifth child, Penina threw herself at her feet and begged for compassion, and they lived."

That Hannah ultimately gave birth to five children is stated explicitly in the text, in Samuel I 2:19-21:

> His mother would make him [Samuel] a small jacket and bring it to him from year to year when she came up with her husband to slaughter the annual offering. And Eli would bless

Elkana and his wife and say, "May God give you children from this woman," because of the request that he [Elkana] requested from God, and they returned to his [Elkana's] place. For God remembered Hannah and she conceived and she bore three sons and two daughters, and the lad Samuel grew up with God [i.e., with Eli in the Tabernacle in Shiloh].

Hannah's story has a happy ending. But we don't want to just skip to the end—we still want to study Hannah's story to elucidate prayer.

Before we do that, though, let's not leave Penina on such a sour note.

Another Explanation for Penina's Behavior

You didn't think there could be a positive slant on this one, did you? But there is.

Let's look carefully at the passage that describes Penina's taunting. There are a few odd features.

"And her adversary would anger her; she would also anger her in order to enrage her, *because God had closed her womb*. And she would do this year after year *whenever they would go up to the house of God*; she would anger her in this way, and she would cry and not eat." (Samuel I 1:6-7.)

Do you notice any oddities? I tried to drop some hints with my added emphases.

According to the omniscient narrator,[7] Penina was trying to make Hannah upset *because* God closed Hannah's womb. Why?

Another point: notice when Penina would taunt Hannah. I imagine they must have lived fairly close together.[8] There were probably endless opportunities for this kind of torment. Why did it happen only when they would go to the house of God? Was this due to practical constraints, i.e. this was the only time they saw each other? If that fact alone explains the timing of the taunts, why would the text go out of its way to record that arbitrary fact? Who cares? Or might there be another reason?

Add these little questions together and they suggest a different slant to the story—that Penina had noble intentions.[9] She hoped that her teasing would inspire Hannah to pray for a child. That would explain why the text emphasizes that Penina angered Hannah every year specifically when they went to the house of God.

So beneath the plain meaning of the story we have uncovered the potential implication that Penina was trying to help. We also have the underlying hint that she was punished for it (granted, that's a lot of subtext).

A deduction is screaming out at us here, and I won't resist it, although the point isn't directly related to infertility.

The interpretation that Penina meant well, but was punished anyway, expresses clear opposition to the philosophy "the ends justify the means." After all, Penina's plan worked! Hannah, in terrible pain, pours her heart out before God, and God responds! Would Hannah's prayer have been effective if Penina hadn't goaded her? (Stay tuned—hopefully we will soon gather enough information to answer that question.)

And yet, Penina suffers consequences. She had no right to inflict that kind of pain on Hannah, no matter how good her intentions. We have no right to put people through pain in order to refine their character. We have no right to design crucibles for other people. Leave that to the Ultimate Silversmith, who will "sit refining and purifying silver." (Malachi 3:3.)

Penina's Women's Intuition

Chazal give us examples of the kinds of things Penina would do:[10] In the morning she would wake up and say to Hannah, "Oh, you don't have to get up and get your children ready for school." At midday, she would say: "Oh, you don't have to wait for your children to come home."

When they were sitting down to eat, she would say in front of Hannah to Elkana: "I need another portion for this son; this son didn't get his portion yet."

This goading was designed to pour salt on the wound, to intensify the emptiness that Hannah was already feeling at those times. The times of day when you know that other mothers are tending to their children—and you aren't—are difficult. There's nothing like getting your nose rubbed in it to magnify your misery. And Penina's chatter in front of Hannah about feeding her children is a masterful stroke of classic passive aggression. Without doing anything overt at all, she calls Hannah's attention to the fact that she, Penina, nourishes her children, while Hannah can't help but notice that she herself has no one to nourish. If Penina had noble intentions, she also had a genius for calculating the perfect shot that would send Hannah sobbing.

I mean, all it takes is one social event where I see three pregnant women and two fussing over their infants and I'm crying. No one has to say anything hurtful to me at all!

Whereas I sit sniffling in the powder room, and complain later to my husband, Hannah did something a little more practical with her crying. Let's take a close look at her inspiring (and successful!) example.

The Vow

What is prayer? How does it work? Can I increase my chances of having my prayers answered?

We all have a sense of what prayer is and how it works. On the most basic level, prayer is asking God for something. Let's see if we can flesh it out by taking a closer look at Hannah's prayer. Samuel I 1:10-12:

> And she was bitter of spirit and she prayed on God and she cried greatly. And she vowed a vow and she said, "God of Hosts, if you see the affliction of your maidservant and you remember me and don't forget your maidservant and give your

maidservant male offspring, then I will give him to God all the days of his life, and a razor will not come to his head." And it was as she increased praying before God, that Eli watched her mouth.

We only get a taste of the words that Hannah used. The text says that she prayed and cried greatly, then it cites the vow, and then it says she increased prayer. But what did she say after her vow? Her prayer must have included other things besides her vow.

There are a few more details that can be gleaned from the rest of the story:

> And Hannah was *speaking to her heart: just her lips were moving, and her voice wasn't audible;* and Eli thought she was drunk. And Eli said to her, "How long will you be drunk? Remove your wine from upon you!" And Hannah answered and said, "No, my master, I am a *bitter-spirited woman* and I have not had wine or strong drink, and I have *poured out my soul before God*. Don't consider your maidservant a base woman because *it is out of my great grievance and anger* that I have spoken [prayed] until now." And Eli answered and said, "Go in peace, and may the God of Israel grant your request that you have asked from him." (Samuel I 1:13-17.)

Keep those highlighted phrases in mind; we'll be using them to weave together a concept of prayer (maybe fold down the corner of the page).

For now, I have a few questions about Hannah's vow.

How does a vow fit in to the idea of prayer? Why is Hannah making this vow and how does it help?

Is Hannah making a deal with God? What can you offer God? He doesn't lack anything. What does He need your son for? How would promising your son to God convince (so to speak) Him to give you a son?

I'm also very interested in Hannah's crying. Is crying a byproduct of prayer, something that happens during prayer, or an essential feature of prayer?

Hannah provides one example of prayer. Let's investigate an additional example. Let's take a look at Moses' prayers.

---

[1] Perhaps you are familiar with the experiment that showed that the pupils of all women tend to dilate when they are shown pictures of babies, whether or not the women are mothers, whereas when the same pictures are shown to men, only the pupils of the fathers tend to dilate.

[2] Radak and Metzudas Dovid 1:9.

[3] Notice how Malbim addressed our earlier question. We said that having a husband is different than having a child. Elkana addressed the area of overlap: someone to help her.

[4] Eleanor Roosevelt.

[5] Metzudas Dovid, Samuel I 2:1.

[6] Radak and Rashi, Samuel I 2:5.

[7] Who was actually Samuel, who later became a prophet.

[8] Remember that, according to Jewish law, Elkana had to provide separate households for them.

[9] The Talmud brings up that possibility, Baba Basra 16a.

[10] Ishei Hatanach, pg. 364.

Chapter XIII

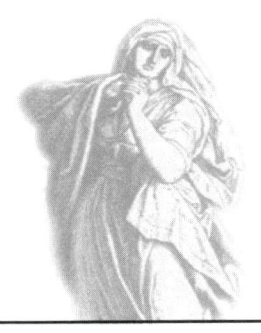

The Power of Prayer

Back to the Pentateuch

I'm going back to the Pentateuch, the first five books of the Torah, because all of the concepts in the Prophets and Writings are expansions of concepts in the Pentateuch.

Moses, the greatest prophet that ever lived or will live, prays a number of times. These prayers are recorded for us in the Bible. I hope studying his prayer can shed some light on Hannah's vow. We could look at any number of examples, but I'll just pick one:

> And Moses pleaded before God, his God, and he said, "Why, God, should Your anger flare up against Your nation that You took out of Egypt with great strength and a mighty hand? Why should Egypt talk, saying: 'With evil intent did He take them out, to kill them in the mountains and to annihilate them from the face of the earth.'? Relent from Your flaring anger and reconsider the evil against Your people. Remember Abraham, Isaac, and Israel Your servants, to whom You swore by Yourself, and You told them, 'I will increase your offspring like the stars of the sky, and all of this land of which I spoke I will give to your offspring and it will be their heritage, forever.'" And God reconsidered regarding the evil He declared He would do to His nation. (Exodus 32:11.)

Guess which national sin Moses was pleading for? The sin of the spies? Korach and his rebellion?[1] A quick look at the preceding verses (7-10) tells us:

> God spoke to Moses: "Go, descend, because your nation that you have taken out of the land of Egypt has become corrupt; they have quickly strayed from the path that I have commanded them; that have made for themselves a molten god, and bowed to it and sacrificed to it, and said, 'These are your gods, Israel, that took you out of the land of Egypt.'" And God said to Moses, "I have seen this nation and behold, they are a stiff-necked people. And now, leave Me alone, and My anger will flare up against them, and I'll wipe them out, and I'll make you into a great nation."

Let's take a closer look at Moses' prayer. He basically offers two arguments: first, "what will Egypt say about this?" and second, "you promised the forefathers." Both arguments seem, at first glance... um...how should I put this...weak. Especially "You promised the forefathers." God is not backing out of his promise—Moses is a descendant of the forefathers. Making a nation that descends from him doesn't violate the promise. So what's the line of reasoning?

There's an even bigger question here, and it's not just about Moses' prayer. In fact, it's a problem with prayer altogether.

How do you make an argument to God? Do you think He doesn't know what you are contending? Of course He knows; He knows everything. So if God already knows your argument, hasn't He already thought through the issues, and *still* decided to go ahead with His decision?

We have said that God lets the laws of nature do their stuff unless there is a reason not to. We could posit that, by respectfully asking God to intervene, our prayer provides the necessary reason. But that doesn't answer the question: why should my prayer change anything?

Whatever argument I muster, God already knows it. Is this a game? Are the rules of the game that unless I go through the motions of formally submitting a request, God won't grant it?

Let's backtrack a little. Moses comes up with an argument or two. Is that prayer? I thought prayer is more like "Please, please, please don't destroy Your nation." Granted, Moses did include a request, I don't mean to minimize that. The element of request is a very important part of prayer. But what's with making a whole case? Isn't prayer just about pleading? What is the point of defending your request and showing God why it makes sense to grant it?

And craziest of all—it worked! Moses apparently made a good case for the continued existence of the nation, because God agreed! But what was actually changed by the prayer? Didn't God have those very same facts *before* Moses voiced the prayer?

My point is not to analyze the specifics of Moses' argument, but I think we can deduce from this example the general concept of *presenting a logical argument in prayer*. If we can untangle that, we'll make strides toward understanding prayer.

How a Logical Argument Works

At first glance, it seems that a logical argument shouldn't help at all. As we said, surely God knows the argument already; is He just making us go through the motions?

There must be something satisfying about the "God is out to get us/God makes us jump through hoops for His own amusement" paradigm; so many of our questions seem to come from this worldview. We think God is out to get us because part of every human being firmly believes, "the entire universe is designed to satisfy ME." I'm sure you don't need a news flash to remind you that this is actually not the case. Things don't go our way, and we sometimes get frustrated. When we get angry, we may even believe the universe (or its designer, i.e., God) is personally thwarting us. We think He gets a big kick out of frustrating us. This is just another way of making it all about ME. Granted, it's a less pleasant way, but at least it's still about ME.

So, to get back to our question—is there actually a point to us praying, to making the request and the logical argument?

Yes; this concept is perfectly in step with everything we've been saying about divine intervention. You see, prayer and stimulating divine intervention are not two separate activities. Isn't prayer just a request for divine intervention? Prayer works the same way that getting God to intervene does.

Let's review. God never changes, no matter what. However, if *we* change, then God relates to us differently. We've discussed some of the different ways we can change. One is by becoming more sensitive to the values and desires that we hold, which leads to an increased awareness of the blind spots that those values and desires can cause when we're raising a child. To put it more generally, unconscious values and desires can cause blind spots in any area where we have to make a decision. To construct a logical argument for the purposes of bringing it to God in prayer, we have to think through carefully: what is important to us and why? Those values, desires, and reasons for them—all those things that go into building a logical argument— are they sound and worthy?

This process of increasing our self-awareness through building a logical argument changes us. It prevents us from being blindly compelled by motivations we aren't aware of; we can make decisions with more knowledge of the factors that drive us.

And infertility (or any type of pain) brings about another change. It pushes us to confront our unspoken feeling that we are entitled to certain things. I have to look at my expectations, look at the reality, and deal with any discrepancies. The struggle between what we want and what we have changes us and challenges our expectations. It shatters illusions and fantasies. Actually, strange as it may sound, it's liberating to be freed of illusions and fantasies. When we get rid of the distraction of what we *wish* would happen, we can devote our full attention to what's *actually happening* instead.

If we can get up after being knocked down by the pain and disappointment, we will be stronger, wiser, and have clearer vision.

These changes may make us worthy of divine intervention. If not, at least we have benefited from the process of refinement, as silver loses its dross when purified by fire.

So the answer to our question about "why pray if it doesn't change God?" is that prayer doesn't change God, but it can change us.

The Power of Prayer

Prayer can change us. It's an amazing thought. I stand before God, I say some things, and I walk away a different person.

But how?

Know Before Whom You Stand

If I'm praying, but I'm imagining that God is my desktop computer, or a flower, is what I'm doing really prayer?

It's basic, it's obvious, but it's fundamental. You have to know whom you're praying to.

It's actually not that easy. People picture a man with a flowing white beard in the sky. God is not physical; any visual or mental image is automatically inaccurate. That deep, baritone voice from *The Ten Commandments* was an actor.

Okay—the guy in charge; the guy running things. Wrong! The Creator is not a "guy." There is no human who is running things. The being? The force? The existence? Now you're closer.

Hannah Did This

There's a rather bizarre phrase that I glossed over earlier, and now is the time to discuss it. Verse 10 says: "And she was bitter of spirit and she prayed *on* God and she cried greatly." Did you notice that weird preposition? Aren't you supposed to pray *to* God? How do you pray *on* God? All of the commentators hasten to assure us that it means *"to God."* But I have to wonder: if that's what the prophet meant, why did he use the word "on?"

The Malbim's explanation illustrates how vital intent is. *"And she prayed on God.* That she prayed with absolute concentration on God *alone."*

On God *alone*. There are a lot of images and all sorts of things that can pop into our heads when we think about God. Accuracy counts here.

Wait 'til you see what Hannah means when she describes God as "Lord of Hosts."

The Request

How does making a request change you?

It's very simple. If I need to ask for something, then I'm acknowledging that I'm not in charge of the distribution system. After all, if I can control whether or not I get it, I don't need to ask. I just go after it. Asking implies, "I need help."

Something interesting happened to me during one of the periods in my life when I was coping with infertility. I had been desultorily praying for a child. When I consulted an infertility specialist, and began the IUI process, the doctor told me confidently, "You will be pregnant on the first try." (Remember, I had "unexplained infertility" and the doctor already knew that both my husband and I had the physical capacity to reproduce.)

So the doctor performed an insemination treatment. That month, I didn't pray very hard to get pregnant. Why didn't I pray more seriously for a child that month? Because I figured the doctor would take care of it. I have confidence in technology and medicine, and if he said he would do it, then I figured he would.

Thirteen days later (I was supposed to take a pregnancy test on the fourteenth day after the insemination) I was staring at blood. Failure! How could this be?

It turned out that I had been briefly pregnant; I had miscarried. I didn't know it at the time, though, and thought that the insemination had failed. In a way it had, if you count success as at least one live child, *but when you can't conceive, any pregnancy, even one that ends in miscarriage, can be considered a step forward.*

This experience really brought home to me that man's technology, no matter how sophisticated, is limited, and that God has an override button. We are just not in control. The next month, I began to seriously study the area of prayer and how it works.

The Logical Argument

Part of prayer is that you *speak* the words (quietly, so that only you hear them). When I make the argument, say it out loud to God, it becomes more real to me. I focus, prioritize, organize my thoughts.

What's the point of making an argument? If prayer is to make a logical argument, but I don't have a logical argument, I just want what I want, should I bother making one? What does that do?

Yes, I should bother because it has an effect on me to assemble a logical argument. In general, I walk around with an unconscious, default attitude: the world is designed to satisfy *me*. But now I have to frame my desires in a less-me-oriented way, taking into account the whole world. If I can do that, it's a statement that I am aware that the world was not created to satisfy me.

I'm not knocking being me-oriented. The problems start when we insist that everything else be oriented toward us occupying the center of our own universe. It's a guaranteed losing proposition to cling to this early-childhood model. My best chance of success in this world is for me to fit myself into it, not to stamp my foot like a sulky child when the world doesn't do what I want.

Summary

We've identified three ways that prayer has an effect on us. One, we focus on the actual Creator, not a projection of our imagination. Two, we acknowledge that we do not have the power to get everything we want. Three, we accept that when our goals and the universe's design butt heads, the universe wins.

---

[1] These episodes are described in Numbers 14:12 and 16:21, respectively.

Chapter XIV

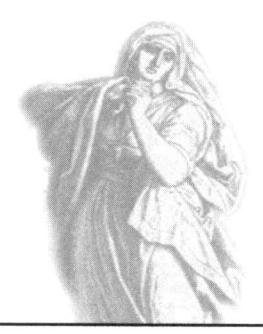

Hannah Continued

The Vow Explained

Let's see if we have enough information now to understand the enigma of Hannah's vow. To recap:

"God of Hosts, if you see the affliction of your maidservant and you remember me and don't forget your maidservant and give your maidservant male offspring, then I will give him to God all the days of his life, and a razor will not come to his head."

First, let's get down the technical meaning of the vow. How do you give a child to God? A mother doesn't have control of her child "all the days of his life." When he gets to a certain age, he takes charge of his life and makes his own decisions. Can his mother's vow be binding on him?

Radak explains: He works in the Temple, like the tribe of Levi, but with a couple of differences. A Levite doesn't start working until he's twenty-five; Samuel worked in the Temple from the time he was very young. (See Samuel I 1:23-28; we also discussed this in the section on Penina.) This is what Hannah meant when she dedicated him to God "all his days." "All his days" refers to his youth, the period of Samuel's life when Hannah made life decisions for him. Therefore she was able to fulfill her vow.

Now to the main problem. How does a vow fit into prayer? Should we be making vows? Is this something that we can still do in the present day? Should we be promising to donate our firstborn children somewhere? The whole idea reminds me of Rumpelstiltskin.

How is the Vow a Logical Argument?

Hannah's vow can be understood as a logical argument that she put before God. We have said that the very formulation of a logical argument helps a person realize, "the universe is not designed purely to gratify me." By constructing an argument, I acknowledge that there may be other factors involved. I try to accommodate myself to those factors.

So what is Hannah's argument?

My understanding of what Hannah is saying is "I realize that You designed human beings in a unique way, God, which indicates that they have a unique purpose. And when You gave babies to mothers, You didn't just have in mind that the purpose was to give mothers pleasure. Human beings can think abstractly; they can think about *themselves*! They can think about a Creator! They can tell the difference between what they *wish* was true and what's *actually* true! God, you made me part of the nation started by Abraham and Sarah, Isaac and Rebecca, and Jacob and Rachel and Leah. The purpose of that nation is to be a shining example of what happens when a human being refines his ability to think abstractly. When a human being lives based on principles of truth and reason, instead of what he *wishes* is true. And God, that nation needs leadership in order for its people to live that kind of a life. And if You give me a son, God, I will not use him as a tool for my own indulgence. I will donate him to serve in Your temple, and I hope that he will ultimately become the kind of leader that can be an inspiration to all of humanity!"

By the way, Samuel grew up to be a leader, a great prophet and judge of the people, just as Hannah had hoped and vowed. In fact, his sense of truth and justice was so strong and clear that the people he led were not quite up to the discomfort that comes with living a life of truth, and they requested a king to lead them rather than a prophet (see Samuel I, 8). God told Samuel, "It is not you whom they have rejected, but it is Me whom they have rejected from reigning over them." (Samuel I, 8:7.)

It's Okay to Want Something

The idea of making a logical argument in the course of prayer is not that there is something inherently bad about wanting something that makes you feel good. It is *not* a tenet of Judaism that it is inherently necessary or beneficial to sacrifice your own desires.

The only consideration is what works and what doesn't, i.e., what is true and what is not. The theory is that since the world is not designed around me, working within the design has a better chance of being successful.

Hannah's Concept Universalized

Hannah's idea applies to everyone. She took what she wanted—to have a child—and fit that personal desire into an objective reason why she should have a child. Then she designed a situation that would help her to internalize this concept. Can you think of a better way to make it crystal-clear to yourself that your child is not a tool for your own pleasure? By "donating" her child, Hannah expressed her grasp of the idea of purposeful human life, that she was not bringing a child into the world merely in order to feel a certain way about herself. This brought her to a level of deserving to have God intervene and grant her a child.

This concept is actually explicit in the Torah.

A Commandment to Donate Your Child?! Yes!

Exodus 13:1,12-13:
> Set aside for Me all firstborn first issue of every womb in the children of Israel, in man and in animal, they are Mine...Set apart every first issue of the womb to God; every first issue of

> your livestock—the males are for God. Every first issue donkey, you should redeem with a lamb or a kid [*and sacrifice it, since a donkey can't be sacrificed*]...And you shall redeem *every human firstborn among your sons.*

Numbers gives us a little more detail, in the section where it describes the various gifts to the priests who work in the Temple and the tithes to the Levites; these "public servants" are not allotted a portion of land with which they can support themselves, so they have to be sustained by the people.

Here is a paraphrase of Numbers 18:15-18:
> Every first issue of a womb of any flesh that they offer to God, whether man or beast, shall be yours [*the priest*]. However, surely redeem the firstborn of man, and the firstborn of a non-kosher animal you shall redeem. The redeeming value is 5 silver shekels. But the firstborn of a cow or sheep or goat you shall not redeem; you shall sacrifice them and eat the meat.[1]

So those are the facts: all firstborns are donated to God, even firstborn humans. However, since we don't go in for human sacrifice, parents are supposed to redeem their firstborn son. This is called *pidyon haben*, still practiced today among many Jews. A mother's firstborn male child is redeemed by paying a *cohen* (any male descended from Aaron the original priest) the equivalent of 5 pieces of silver.

You may be wondering, "what does this have to do with Hannah?" *The Book of Education* provides this insightful analysis of Commandment 18 in *Parshas Bo* (paraphrased slightly):
> This commandment is for a person to realize that everything is His, and that man only has in the world what God in His kindness gave to him. This is the way he understands this: after the person makes a lot of effort and puts in a lot of energy and work in his situation, when he finally gets to the

point of fruition, and the first that he produces is as dear to him as the apple of his eye, he immediately gives this first produce to God and empties his possession from himself and enters it into the possession of his Creator.

The moment a human being finally produces, after so much effort, the moment when his efforts will be rewarded with the sweet satisfaction of success, there is danger—danger of arrogance, danger of mistaken conceit. It is tempting to believe, "I am entirely responsible for my own success!"

To some extent, it's true—I carried out my responsibilities and I get some credit for the results. Without my own effort, I would produce no product. If I don't plant, I grow no crops. If I don't work, I don't bring home a paycheck.

But I'm not the *only* one responsible. There are lots of factors that I can't control. Sure, I planted the seeds, but I do not govern the rain and the sun and I can't prevent tomato hornworm infestations. And if I don't keep in mind the limitations to my role, I may well become arrogant. Clearly, even with my best efforts, all those other factors have to be in place for my crops to succeed.

The same feeling applies to having children. You put in so much energy and effort that when you finally succeed, it's easy to ignore all the other factors that made it possible. To remind us of those factors, we "pay" God for the baby. This payment helps us to remember that we don't really own this child, that we are not the only cause of its existence.

Hannah truly understood this. Voicing her prayer and vow before God concretized this concept from an idea inside her head to a reality in her heart and mind. She took her desire for a child and aligned it with the design of the universe. God heeded her prayer.

---

[1] Some sacrifices are totally burnt, and some are partially burnt and the rest eaten by the priests and the person who brings the sacrifice.

Chapter XV

How Does Prayer Work?

The Gates of Tears Are Never Closed

The more we can learn about how prayer works, the more chance of our prayers being answered. Let's explore some more concepts of prayer, starting with the crying.

"And she was bitter of spirit, and she prayed on God, and she cried greatly." (Samuel I 1:10.)

"I am a woman of aggrieved spirit...and I poured my soul before God." (Samuel I 1:15.)

"The Gates of Tears are never closed." (Malbim[1] on "And she cried greatly.")

How Does Crying Help?

How does crying help our prayers get answered? At first glance, this doesn't seem to fit what we've said about prayer so far. In fact, it poses a problem.

Take a flesh-and-blood person. Make a request in front of him. The request is so important to you that you start crying as you plead your case.

How does the crying work in that case? You stir a feeling of compassion in the person, and he's moved to help you. You've elicited an emotional response.

That doesn't work for God. What would we be saying if it did? That you can manipulate God? That God didn't necessarily intend to grant your request, but when you started crying, His heart melted?

That approach does not hold up to scrutiny, because what changed? Nothing! You are not more deserving of your request being granted because you're crying; you didn't present new information. If crying is supposed to show God how much the request means to you—He's omniscient; He already knows that!

The idea of God acquiescing more readily to more emotional requests smacks of parents caving in to their children's requests because it breaks their hearts to see them cry. True, it is a tempting quality to attribute to God—that He's a loving parent who hurts when His children hurt, therefore, because He can't tolerate the pain, the gates of tears are never closed.

But this view would put God at the mercy of His emotions. Him and His emotions—oh no, parts! Plus not very omnipotent. Not even very good parenting, if you rephrase it as "parents caving in to their children's demands and tantrums because it breaks their hearts to see them cry."

Chazal's statement, "I (God) am with you in your trouble (Exodus 3:2, Rashi)" does not mean that God makes decisions He wouldn't otherwise make because of the discomfort of the pain.

Let's see if there's another way to understand this.

Crying Can't Change God; It Must Change Me

This leads us back to our basic approach. We've said it before: prayer doesn't change God. It changes me, which may trigger divine intervention.

There is just one problem. Crying doesn't really change a person. I may feel temporarily relieved, or cleansed, or exhausted, but permanent change comes from new insight, new understanding. How can tears provide that insight?

Standing before God

It's not enough to cry; crying alone doesn't have a lasting effect on us. But crying in front of God does.

Maimonides says: What does it mean to concentrate (during prayer)? A person should turn his heart from all thoughts and see himself as if he is standing before the Divine Presence.[2]

What does it mean to "see yourself as if you're standing before God"? You're always before Him. That's what omniscience is all about!

Obviously, the seeing is not from God's perspective. *See yourself.* It means in *your* mind, in *your* conscious awareness. Prayer is the experience of standing before your Creator.

Crying before God

Why are the gates of tears never closed? How does crying before God affect you?

You cry out of desperation. You cry when the feeling sweeps over you that you cannot get what you want. You want it so badly, yet it's just not up to you. You cry out of helplessness, frustration, impotence. You can't get it for yourself, and you beg someone who can to help you.

And in essence, that's what prayer is. Prayer is about the true recognition of your place in the scheme of things. No human experience captures that recognition more powerfully than standing in front of our Creator, acknowledging by our tears that we realize that we do not even have enough control to fulfill our own needs.

Hannah's Threat

While you are throwing yourself on God's mercy, begging and pleading for what you want, why not threaten Him as well? Ridiculous, right?

Threatening God seems counterproductive to getting what you want. But that's what Hannah does.

Talmud Brachos 31b comments on the verse, "If you see [*Ra'oh tir'eh*] the affliction of your maidservant" (1:11) as follows: "If you see, then good. And if not, you will see. I will go and hide before my husband, and they will feed me the *Sotah* waters, and you won't make your Torah a fraud as it says, 'If she is innocent she will have children.'"

The basis of this exegesis is the double wording of *Ra'oh tir'eh* (literally, "if you see, you will see"). Often the text uses a repeated root in different forms for emphasis ("Go, you will go" means "definitely go"), which helps to express the plain meaning. But Chazal saw this sort of double use of a word as giving a hint to deeper meaning, and used these oddities of word usage as openings to express additional concepts.

In this case, the plain meaning is that the double language is the beginning of Hannah's vow. "If you see my affliction, and give me a son, then I will…" But Chazal use the subtlety of the double language to communicate another aspect of prayer. "If you see" my affliction, and give me a son, then fine. If not, "you will see" what I do.

The threat itself is absurd. Job 35:6-7: "If you are righteous, what do you give Him; or what does He receive from your hand? If you sinned, what do you achieve against Him? And if your sins are a lot, what do you do to Him?" God designed a system to benefit man. Hannah would only harm herself by becoming a Sotah.

What's a Sotah?

An entire tractate of the Talmud is devoted to the *Sotah*; many of the details are not recorded in the written law. (see Numbers 5:11-31.)

The entire set of laws is called the "law of jealousies." (Numbers 5:29.) These laws apply when a husband is overcome with jealousy because he has found out that his wife was alone with another man—not just any man, but a man whom he had specifically warned her not to be alone with. (Are you getting a feel for the state of this marriage?) Now the husband suspects her of committing adultery.

If the wife admits to the adultery, the couple can get a nice quiet divorce and the Sotah laws are not relevant. But what happens when she denies that she commited adultery and she wants to keep the marriage intact? Then she becomes a Sotah.

This dramatic procedure is designed to prove the Sotah's innocence or guilt, that is whether she is telling the truth when she denies having committed adultery. She goes to the Temple and takes an oath that she has not committed adultery. The priest warns her that her stomach will burst if she's lying. She acknowledges her awareness of the danger. The priest writes down the oath (which includes God's name) and erases it by dissolving it in water mixed with dirt from the floor of the Temple (by the way, the commandment that it is forbidden to erase God's name is suspended in this case). She drinks the water. If she is guilty of adultery, her stomach bursts and she dies. (Remember, if she knows she is guilty, she has the option of admitting to adultery and accepting a divorce without going through this process.) And if her stomach does not burst and she remains alive, "then she will be proven innocent, and she will bear seed [*have a child*]." (Numbers 5:28.)

Let's take a closer look at Hannah's apparent plan. If God doesn't give her a child, then she will scheme to be brought in front of the priest as a Sotah. Remember the great love between Hannah and her husband Elkana? This plan would seem to involve Hannah's causing her husband to be suspicious of her, and allowing herself to be caught alone with a man that Elkana specifically mistrusts her with. Although she wouldn't commit adultery, she would still have had to compromise her marriage and her modesty. She would have had to be willing to pay this price in order to reap the benefit of being proven innocent—to "bear seed."

Do you think Hannah had this in mind when she made her threat to God? What do you think of the wisdom of such a plan? Besides the damage Hannah would be risking to her marriage, would this scheme really work? The procedure for judging a Sotah was designed to call in divine assistance to help stabilize a troubled marriage when both people sincerely want to make it work. It involves humiliation to both spouses. If Hannah would go through a manufactured charade of the procedure, attempting to take advantage of a technicality (the promise that at the end she would bear a child), would it have produced an effective magical formula for bearing a child?

That doesn't make sense. The promise of a child to a Sotah whose innocence has been proven is the promise of divine intervention for two spouses who have undergone a certain painful and demanding experience and come to a new understanding of what it means to build a home together. A child is a natural outgrowth of that harmony; God intervenes to make it happen. How could the artificial invoking of the procedure possibly work for Hannah? And at what price?

The real challenge here is to understand how this element fits in to the idea of prayer. When we understand that, we'll know what Hannah meant when she uttered her threat.

My Story

I mentioned earlier that I began studying Hannah's story because her success intrigued me and I wanted to know her secret. The month before I began studying her story, I had unsuccessfully attempted Intra-Uterine Insemination (IUI). The whole IUI process was difficult for me. I was squeamish about injecting myself, so a relative who was a nurse gave me the shots. Every day I toyed with the idea of giving myself the shot, but I knew I would spend all day worrying that I might have done it wrong. I reacted badly to the medication, and my legs were sore from the injections and it hurt when I walked. My ovaries got hyper-stimulated and swelled up painfully. And on and on.

A friend of mine went through this procedure four times before she conceived. The very fact that other people do put themselves through this multiple times makes me realize that perhaps I'm more than a tad spoiled about tolerating discomfort. I was seriously thinking twice even about doing IUI a second time. In any case, I had to take a month off to let my ovaries recuperate from the over-stimulation. The doctor asked us if we wanted to go on the pill, so that we could cut down the time until we could climb back on the baby-making bandwagon to a mere twenty-one days. My husband and I looked at each other and said, "No, we'll go natural this month and see what happens (ha, ha)." My husband was definitely gung-ho to try again. Easy for him to say; they weren't *his* ovaries. I was less enthusiastic to try again; my legs and emotions and ovaries were all protesting loudly in chorus.

Going through the IUI had a profound effect on me. I had to grapple with the physical discomfort, the stress of the blood tests and the sonograms and the incessant visits to the doctor. But perhaps more important, I had to come to terms with the fact that life wasn't going my way, and the only way to get what I wanted was via a great deal of inconvenience, discomfort, and angst. The whole situation aroused a lot of feelings about my sense of self, my wants, and my self-image.

As often happens when a painful process churns up strong feelings, I did not rush to embrace these insights about myself. I ignored them as best as I could, and when that month's introspection was over, I was relieved.

The next month I had to decide whether to repeat the IUI procedure. I was torn. I knew that I had pushed away a number of perceptions about myself, and that they were hovering in the periphery of my consciousness, waiting for a new round of pain to force me to deal with them. I knew that sometimes a person escapes a situation before he has had the chance to fully explore what it can teach him. However, though pain can transform a person, does anybody in their right mind deliberately seek out pain?

This was one of the questions I had when I began studying the story of Hannah.

Prayer of Desperation: Laying It on the Line before God

Hannah's threat intrigued me. She was driven to pray by Penina's taunts. When she prays her song of thanks, the first reason she offers for her praise is "My heart rejoices with God, my horns have been raised up through God [*i.e., she can hold up her head in pride or she can defend herself*], my mouth is opened wide against my enemies, for I rejoice in Your salvation." (Samuel I 2:1.) Shouldn't her primary motivation to offer praise be to give thanks for the child she has borne, the child she so desperately wanted? Yet the first thing that she mentions is the relief of her humiliation.

We can see from this example that the prime motivation for seeking God's help is for relief from pain. A person in pain who throws himself on God's mercy is opening himself up to understanding the primary relationship between Creator and created: dependency.

I understood Hannah's threat in this framework. Perhaps Hannah was throwing herself on God's mercy. Perhaps this threat was Hannah's way of stating before God, "This is how desperate I am. This is how much pain I feel. I am even considering putting my marriage at risk and jeopardizing my relationship to You because I want a child so badly. This is what's going through my head. I'm desperate! Help me!"

Hannah's threat seemed to me to be a statement of desperation before God. When you stand before God and lay everything on the line, precisely expose before God your emotional wretchedness and desperation, it crystallizes your relationship with Him. I, the petitioner, have to be completely honest before the One who has the power to grant.

Application

It worked for Hannah, so I hoped it would work for me. I mapped out my prayer. Using what I gleaned from Hannah's prayer, I planned to stand before God and request a child based on my understanding of my role and my purpose as a human being that He created. Then I planned to beg shamelessly, to open my heart and fully express how painful it is for me, how it hurts so much and how I want the pain to end. How much I hated going through the treatments. How much I just wanted the pain to stop.

I would do this knowing that it would heighten my awareness of my vulnerability and powerlessness, my inability to rescue myself from this situation. It would bring home to me my place in the universe vis-à-vis God.

That month the doctor also sent me for an uncomfortable and invasive test called a histosalpingogram, for which they insert a catheter and inject dye into your uterus. This test reveals any mechanical blockages that may be preventing conception. Even if there are no serious blockages that would need to be removed via surgery (or worse, that are untreatable), the dye that is flushed through the system can "clean you out."

And...

That was the month I conceived my daughter Chana (Hebrew for Hannah).

---

[1] The Malbim is quoting the Talmud here (Bava Metzia 59a and Berachos 32b): Rabbi Eliezer said, "From the day the Temple was destroyed, the gates of prayer were closed...And even though the gates of prayer were closed, the gates of tears were not closed."

[2] Laws of Prayer 4:16.

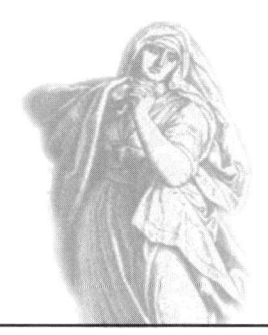

Chapter XVI

When Prayer Isn't Answered

What happens when our prayers aren't answered? What if we think carefully, line up our desires with the design of the world, build a logical argument explaining how our desires harmonize with God's will, recognize that God is in control—and our prayers *still* aren't answered?

Before we start this discussion, let's put our expectations and desires in perspective: we get many benefits in this world without needing to earn them. Air to breathe, water to drink, and even food is fairly plentiful on the planet (and many countries even have climate control, public transportation, and TV entertainment in your own home). What we are asking for in our prayers is often "extra." King David, in Psalms 8:5, expresses amazement that God would intervene on man's behalf: "What is man, that You remember him? And the son of man, that You pay attention to him?" So we are presuming a lot by believing that we deserve to have our prayers answered—that it is only fair that we get what we want.

But we still try. It may take a long time for our prayers to be answered–even years. We may not know for sure whether or not a prayer will ever be answered.

"Not Now"

Thinking back to Rachel, her prayers were answered after many years. She used the fertility drugs of the time, the *dudaim*, and still it took years; Leah had two more sons and a daughter in the interim—at least 27 months elapsed—before Rachel gave birth to her first child. *Years* after Rachel used the *dudaim* and gave her handmaiden to her husband, "God remembered Rachel and listened to her and opened her womb." (Genesis 30:22.) Sometimes it feels like our prayers aren't being answered, but it may be that God will answer them eventually, according to His own calculation.

Sometimes the Answer is *No*

But as a friend once told me, "Sometimes the answer is *no*." We don't like this answer. It causes some people to question whether God even exists. It may be easier to assume that the world runs according to fixed laws than to believe in a non-responsive God, or in a God that responds, but not to me.

So not all prayers are answered, though they may be offered with all appropriate intention and thought. Even Moses, the paradigm of the petitioner, got an unequivocal response in Deuteronomy 3:23: The answer is *no*, and don't nag me about it any more.

> And I begged God at that time saying, "God, Lord—You began to show Your servant Your greatness and Your strong hand; who is like God in the heavens and the earth that can do like Your deeds and Your strength? Please, let me cross and see the good land on the other side of the Jordan, this good mountain and the Lebanon." And God got angry at me on your behalf, and He didn't listen to me, and God said to me, "It's enough; don't talk to Me about this anymore."

Many of the laws of prayer are learned from this particular one, considered a model prayer—a prayer that was refused![1] What good is a prayer that doesn't work?

It is painful and disappointing to make a sincere effort at prayer, and still have your prayer go unfulfilled.

Once, in my fourth month of pregnancy, after other pregnancies had terminated in miscarriage, I was put on bed-rest for three weeks in an attempt to sustain the pregnancy. The day after I took to bed, I started to feel the baby kick. A few days earlier, the sonogram had told me it was a boy. I so hoped that my prayers would allow me to carry this son to term.

For three weeks, in bed, I planned and made my daily prayers. I spent a lot of time thinking about what I wanted to ask, trying to expand my personal desire for my son to survive into an objective framework. I tried to refine my own understanding of my purpose in life and how it would relate to raising this child (you have a lot of time to think when you're confined to bed); I thought at length about my lack of control over this situation, and my dependence on my creator. I begged for compassion.

Then my waters broke. I had just begun my fifth month. There was no chance of the baby's surviving.

Prayer and Heartache

The Talmud (Brachos 32b) says:
> Rabbi Yochanan said: "Whoever prays at length and has intent will end up having heartache, as it says (Proverbs 13:12), 'Hope deferred makes the heart sick'"... Rabbi Chama said in the name of Rabbi Chanina: If a person sees that he prayed and wasn't answered, let him go back and pray again as it says (Psalms 27:14), 'Hope to God, be strong and let your heart take courage, and hope to God.'"

The end of this discussion is inspiring, but the beginning is difficult. Why heartache? Isn't intent a good thing when we pray? Certainly intent is one of the necessary ingredients; prayer without intent and concentration isn't even prayer!

Rashi explains what type of intent this means: "He expects that his request will be fulfilled because he prayed with proper intent. In the end, when his request is not fulfilled, it will end up being 'a hope pushed away' [a more literal translation of *a hope deferred*] and for nothing. And it is a heartache when a person has an expectation and his desire doesn't come to pass."

I can relate to the heartache part; I'm sure you can too. But isn't prayer all about making a request? Prayer seems like an ironic construction: make a request, but don't expect even a properly-made request to be granted. Then why bother?

What is Prayer Really For?

"God is close to all who call to Him—to all that call to Him in truth." (Psalms 145:18.) I used to think that meant that God will answer anyone who calls out sincerely. But then how can it be that even Moshe Rabbeinu, master of all prophets, called out and was told "no"? In what sense can we understand the idea that God is close to those who call to Him in truth?

Read the verse carefully. It does not guarantee that God will grant the request of every true prayer. What it does guarantee is that God is close to anyone who calls out to Him in truth. This is the true measure of the success of prayer.

A successful prayer is one that brings the petitioner closer to God. The method that we use to get closer to God is to stand before Him and make requests. The goal is not to have our request *answered*; the goal is to call out to God in truth. It seems odd, but the main object of the request is not to have it fulfilled—the point of prayer is that making a request clarifies our understanding of God and His universe.

On the most basic level, I, the petitioner, request from God, the grantor. Making the request renders clear to me God's role and my role in our relationship—who is in charge and who needs help. This is the fundamental relationship between God and me: Creator and created.

The specifics of my request and how I present it can bring me closer to God. My request can help me understand how God's world is designed and how I fit into it. The more I appreciate this, the closer I am to God.

That is why Moses' prayer, an unanswered prayer, is an illustration for us. Any time we enter the arena of prayer, we have the opportunity to develop increasingly profound insight into God's design of the world. Even when our prayers go unanswered, God, in his compassion, wants us to benefit from the process of prayer itself. Sincere prayer is never wasted.

When we pray, we try to understand God's design and present an argument that shows how the design will be enhanced by the granting of our desires. We hope that God will heed our prayer. But expecting our prayer to be granted is asking for disappointment. We can't be confident that God will respond to our prayer because that is not the objective of prayer.

The opportunity God gives us when we pray is *not* to get what we want. Prayer gives us the chance to creatively explore our relationship with God and our place in his world. If we have done that, even when we do not get what we asked for, we can be confident that our prayer has achieved its true objective.

---

[1] Talmud Brachos 32a.

Chapter XVII

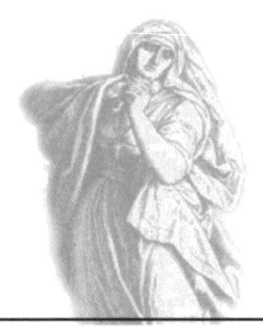

King David and Infant Loss

Each time a Matriarch becomes pregnant, the Biblical text describing her life testifies, "And she conceived, and she gave birth [in Hebrew, *VaTahar VaTeled*]." When I was growing up, I always wondered why the Torah made a point of using both terms, over and over again. I took the usual course of events for granted—first she conceived, then she gave birth. Why recite all the steps?

Events in my own life have given me a new appreciation for the phenomenon of "she conceived and she gave birth"—"*VaTahar VaTeled*." Conception is not always followed by successful, live birth.

During the years I was trying to conceive Chana, I had two early-pregnancy miscarriages. Since Chana's birth, I have had two losses, both in the fifth month of pregnancy. I had felt the babies moving inside me for a number of weeks before these later-pregnancy losses.

King David dealt not with pregnancy loss, but with infant loss. He has an unexpected approach to loss—an approach that the people around him find backwards. We will see that King David's clear understanding and acceptance of the design of the universe changes the nature of his emotional reactions. A person who spends his whole life trying to fit into God's design has very different emotions from those of a person who spends his energy fighting God's design.

David's Story

Do you know the famous story of David and Bathsheba (*Batsheva*, in the original Hebrew)? While his army is away at war, King David sees Bathsheba bathing on a nearby rooftop. He falls in lust and takes her for himself, though she is married to Uriah, one of David's army officers. When Bathsheba gets pregnant, King David attempts a cover-up by bringing the officer home, but Uriah refuses to be intimate with his wife while his soldiers are out fighting for their lives. King David orders his general to place Uriah in the thick of battle, where he is killed, and King David marries Bathsheba.

Due to legal technicalities adamantly detailed by the commentators, King David committed neither adultery nor murder. However, though King David did not technically violate a single law, the divine denunciation is clear: "And the thing that David did was bad in the eyes of God." (Samuel II 11:27.)

King David's confrontation of his errors is heroic, and deserves study as a paradigm for admitting our mistakes. Now we are going to look at what happened after that.

The narrative continues in Samuel II 12:13-23:

> And David said to Nathan (the prophet), "I have sinned to God." And Nathan said to David, "Also, God removed your sin—you will not die. However, since you greatly degraded the enemies of God (*a euphemism for the honor of God*) in this matter, also the child that is born to you will surely die."

> And Nathan went to his house, and God smote the child that the wife of Uriah bore to David, and he got very sick. And David beseeched God for the child, and David fasted, and as often as he went in, he lay all night on the ground. And the elders of his household stood beside him to lift him from the ground, but he wouldn't, and he wouldn't have even a little bread with them.

And on the seventh day the boy died, and David's servants were afraid to tell him that the child died because they said, "Look, while the boy was alive we spoke to him and he wouldn't listen to us. How can we tell him the boy died? He might harm himself!" And David saw that his servants were whispering and David understood that the boy was dead. And David said to his servants, "Did the boy die?" and they said, "He died."

And David got up from the ground and he washed and anointed himself and changed his clothing. And he came to the house of God and he bowed, and he came to his house and he requested, and they put for him, bread and he ate. And his servants said to him, "What is this thing that you did? On behalf of the live child, you fasted and cried. And when the boy died, you got up and you ate bread." And he said, "While the boy was still alive, I fasted and I cried; because I said, 'Who knows if God will have mercy on me and the boy might live?' But now, he is dead. Why would I fast—can I bring him back anymore? I go to him [*to the grave, when I die*]¹, but he will not come back to me."

King David's reaction is incomprehensible to the people around him. He spent days crying over his son before the child died, even refusing to be distracted with food. Everyone expected him to react with anguish to his son's death—surely he would be crazed with grief when the child died, given how he had acted before! Instead, though King David had seemed tormented during his son's illness, when the boy died he got up, washed and ate. What explains his behavior? It can't be indifference to the death of his child; his previous intensity rules that out. So what is going on?

The Punishment Factor

Before we answer that, it is important to point out: this is a punishment. As we said earlier, you cannot assume that your situation is a punishment unless a prophet explicitly tells you so, as the prophet Nathan told David; but you also can't rule out the possibility. In our lives today, without any prophets around, we take the route of introspection and try to understand what a tragedy can teach us about ourselves. If this process uncovers sins, distortions in our worldview, or mistakes we have made, the path of repentance is always open to us.

It is a good idea to consult someone you trust to help you differentiate between "sins" and "things I feel guilty about." It may well be that not everything that you feel badly about is genuinely wrong. For example, let's say you have a hard time saying "no" to people. One of your friends constantly takes advantage of this trait, though she never reciprocates. She knows you are up to your elbows cooking dinner to help out a sick neighbor who is supposed to entertain her husband's boss. Still, she asks you to do her a favor—the third one this week—and pick up her brother from the airport.

In a rare moment of strength, you refuse apologetically, but you still feel like a piece of lint. If something bad would then happen to you, would your first thought be that it's a punishment for being a selfish person by saying "no" to a friend?

I can personally testify that all sorts of wacky feelings run through my mind when tragedy hits. I find it very helpful to be reassured that whatever sins I am imagining are not the cause of the misfortune.

God's justice is undoubtedly quite different from the superstitious whims that our creative, guilt-ridden minds attribute to Him. Looking at the issue carefully can actually teach us a lot about the "universes in our own minds," as my theological consultant put it—the hazy ideas that we make up about reward and punishment and how we think God is running, or should be running, the world.

How can you do this? Compare what you fear and imagine to the guidelines that you know, and identify the differences between how you feel the universe is being run and the principles that you can know for sure. And if you really did something that was so awful that it merits serious punishment—it is important to face the truth. You can always, always change. It is terrifying to confront the truth, but what is the alternative? Maimonides says: "When I [God] bring tragedy upon you so that you will repent, if you say that it is a coincidence then this is cruelty that causes you to stick to your evil ways."[2]

A lesson for all of us to keep in mind: King David, knowing from the mouth of a prophet that this was a punishment and that his child would die, *still* tried to change himself and his understanding of the universe so that his child would live. If he thought it was worth a shot, why should we think differently?

David's "Callousness"

We are going to explore the seeming contradiction in King David's reaction to the death of his son. When he "should" be throwing himself on the floor weeping, he calmly gets up instead. When he "should" be too numb to eat, he asks for food; when he "should" be tearing his clothes in grief, he anoints himself and changes into fresh clothing.

It is interesting to note that King David's reaction to this baby's death differs from his reaction to the subsequent deaths of two of his grown sons, Absalom and Amnon. (Yes, King David had a really tough life. Don't he and the Matriarchs and Patriarchs just devastate the myth that those beloved of God lead a charmed life?) According to Jewish law, the guidelines for mourning, which include tearing the clothing to demonstrate grief and a prohibition against washing during the week of mourning, do not apply in the case of the death of an infant younger than one month of age or to a stillbirth.

Radak comments on Samuel II 12:21 that King David considered crying for this baby to be different from the usual crying for someone who dies. "He is not a developed personality[3] where someone would cry about the loss of that particular individual." It's not that King David didn't cry over his losses; he wept for Amnon and Absalom out of his anguish and mourning. He mourned the loss of the sons he had known and with whom he had had relationships, and cried from the anguish he felt at losing them.

Two Types of Cries

Why didn't King David cry when his baby died? How do you not cry when your tiny son dies, especially a son you spent days crying and begging God to save?

The commentators are unanimous. The crying and fasting that the servants thought stemmed from King David's suffering over his son's illness was, in fact, prayer. King David used every available minute pleading for mercy as long as there was still a chance that the boy would survive.

"But now, he is dead. Why would I fast—can I bring him back anymore? I go to him but he will not come back to me." With this simple statement, King David explains why he does not cry. "There is no prayer for the impossible, only for the possible." (Malbim on Samuel II 12:22.)

"Can I bring him back anymore?" The only kind of crying left to King David was an attempt to bring the baby back; cries of prayer were no longer a possibility. And King David ruled out a futile attempt to bring the baby back through crying. "I go to him but he will not come back to me."

The Loss of What Could Have Been

Of course we cry; it's a legitimate reaction. I'm not bringing up the story of King David to tell us not to cry. In fact, miscarriage after treatment for infertility is recognized as causing an even more profound feeling of loss than miscarriage after unassisted conception, because the couple knows they can't "just conceive again," and the effort to conceive has cost them so much, emotionally, physically, even financially.

But, although King David felt anguish and mourning at the loss of his children, he did not mourn his dreams of what might have been.

Every pregnancy carries the hope of a potential life. The longer it continues, the more viable the new life seems, and the more we think of it as real. We become attached to our babies, especially if we feel them move, or see them, or hold them, or—even more wrenching if we lose them later—nurse them. We form relationships with our babies, and who they will become. And these are all things we must mourn. The loss of our hopes, the loss of the images we carry in our hearts of what we would have had. When it's over, we cling to the possibility, the potential that was. But death ends the game. The hopes and dreams that were expressed in this potential life can no longer see fruition. "I go to him, but he will not come back to me."

Why didn't King David cry? Because he wasn't attached to gossamer dreams that, regardless of their prior potential splendor, could no longer come true.

For me, it's a persistent struggle to deal with the reality of my situation. I have thoughts of what "should" be happening, and I get upset that it isn't. I "should" be eight months pregnant now. My son "should" be crawling now. But King David does not dwell in the realm of "should." He lives in the world that exists, not in the world he wishes would exist. When he can change things, he struggles courageously to do so. And when it's over, it is clear to him that the current state of nonexistence of this baby is all that there is.

King David didn't deliberately decide to feel this way. His emotional reaction was a result of his knowledge and understanding. As a leader of the nation founded by Abraham and the Patriarchs and Matriarchs, and following their ideals and principles, he did not live in a world of his own imagination, but bravely lived in the world that God had designed.

May King David's strength and wisdom comfort us as we cry for our lost dreams, and as we shed tears for our babies that we cannot bring back.

---

[1] Metzudas Dovid, Samuel II 12:23.
[2] Paraphrase from Maimonides, Laws of Fasts 1:3.
[3] Literally "*ben da'as*," creature of knowledge.

Chapter XVIII

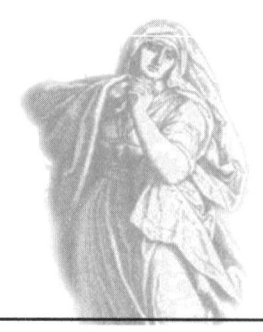

Final Thoughts

I needed a book like this, one that deals with the spiritual aspect of infertility, during my own infertility, and there was none available. Undeniably, it is a painful experience to be unable to give birth to and raise a biological child. But the social aspects, our own narcissism, and our disappointment over shattered dreams serve to magnify and intensify this pain. The experience of pain obligates a person to introspect about his deeds and values. I hope that this book has opened the door for you to explore some of your own expectations and fantasies that might make infertility so painful for you.

I've talked a lot about getting God to intervene, to answer our prayers, to change the laws of nature or to give them a little nudge on our behalf. This is a tricky area, and not scientifically demonstrable because there is no way to know for sure that divine intervention has taken place (unless you have an open-and-shut case like that of Abraham and Sarah, where Sarah conceived after having been post-menopausal for nearly half a century). We *want* God to intervene, but the only way to achieve divine intervention, if at all, is to re-align our expectations with the way the universe actually runs. It's not easy to adjust our expectations. Our best bet is to become more self-aware: what are our expectations, and how do they differ from reality?

The main struggle of human existence is to find a way to swim out of the quagmire of our blind spots and wishes, and see what's actually going on around us. Gaining an understanding of our place in the universe is the greatest reward for having worked through this process. The goal of having a child may not succeed; achieving greater insight is a gift nonetheless.

Isaiah puts it poignantly (56:3-5):
> And let not the barren one say, "Behold, I am a shriveled tree." For thus said God to the barren ones who observe My Sabbaths and choose what I desire, and grasp My covenant tightly: "In my house and within my walls I will give them a place of honor and renown, which is *better than sons and daughters*; eternal renown will I give them, which will never be terminated."

The prophet is referring to a specific type of despondency. A person who can't have children may naturally get depressed about the future, eternity and the lack of continuity through the generations. "What is the point of my life? I'm like a withered tree that can't bear fruit. What is the value of my living a principled life? What does it matter?"

Isaiah is talking about the yearning for immortality, the search for meaning. Without progeny, does life have meaning? Many people talk about how their lives seemed more purposeful once they'd held their newborn babies in their arms. Suddenly, there seemed to be an unbroken line stretching back into the past and forward into the future, generation after generation. Existence suddenly seemed to be much more than just your own individual life. And it's true—there is something "grander than your own life" when you feel yourself to be a link in the chain of humanity stretching between the past and the future.

But when you read this passage from Isaiah, you see that God is communicating a clear and unambiguous principle. The type of eternity that every human being yearns for is not achieved by having children. The most valuable thing that a human being can do is live his own life to the best of his ability. This is how each of us can earn ourselves eternal and interminable honor and renown.

May we merit enough personal growth and insight to find real comfort in this truth.

Meet the Commentators

Here's a bit of biographical information on the commentators that I have quoted throughout the book, arranged in alphabetical order by last name.

Ibn Ezra

Abraham Ibn Ezra is a Spanish scholar who lived from 1089-1167. He was a brilliant grammarian and poet. A major principle that he advocates is that logic is the foundation for the study of the Torah.

Nehama Leibowitz

The most "recent" of the commentators I've quoted (1905-1997), Nehama Leibowitz is famous for her keen analysis of the text and the commentators. Her questions open areas of knowledge. She lived in Jerusalem most of her life. The inscription on her tombstone is simply *Nehama Leibowitz Morah* (teacher).

Maimonides

Moses ben Maimon, or Maimonides, also known as the Rambam (1135-1204), was born in Spain. He wrote a systematic code of all Jewish law, as well as a deeply philosophical treatise *The Guide to the Perplexed* (catchy title, no?). He published a commentary on the entire Mishna in his early twenties (!) and was the physician of the Sultan of Egypt.

Malbim

Meir Leibush ben Yechiel Michel (1809-1879, Eastern Europe) wrote a commentary on the entire Bible, but is used in this book to illuminate the writings of the prophets. He is particularly sensitive to the different nuances in seemingly repetitive, poetic phrases.

Metzudas Dovid

This is the pen name of Rabbi David Altschuler, an eighteenth-century Galician exegete. It means "Tower of David" which King David built and used as part of Jerusalem's defense system (do you see the symbolism?). He is a favorite of mine; I always look to his commentary first to help me untangle the plain meaning of verses from the prophets and writings.

Onkelos

A second century proselyte who converted to Judaism, Onkelos was the nephew of the Roman Emperor. There are a number of stories about his quick thinking in the Talmud, especially how he handled his uncle's attempts to dissuade him from studying. His Aramaic translation of the Bible is usually located right next to the original text.

Radak

Rabbi David Kimchi (1157-1236) was a grammarian from Southern France. I use his commentary on the prophets to gain deeper insight into the text.

Rambam

See "Maimonides," above.

Ramban

Rabbi Moshe ben Nachman (1194-1270) is one of the more voluble commentators. He elucidates areas rather than phrases. He is fascinating in the way he vehemently disagrees with other commentators while still holding them in profound respect.

Rashbam

Rabbi Samuel ben Meir, grandson of Rashi (1085-1174), took his grandfather's love of brevity to a new level in his Bible commentary. His goal was to explain the plain meaning of the text.

Rashi

Rabbi Shlomo Yitzchaki (1040-1105) was a French scholar who commented on almost every single verse in the Torah. (I have seen Rashi's commentary referred to as "the Cliff Notes of the Bible.") On the surface, his commentary seems easy to understand and is the first commentary taught to young children. However, his simplicity is misleading. In some cases he quotes a Talmudic interpretation of a particular verse, while in others he states a more literal explanation. I find his commentary to be one of the most difficult to understand, especially the allegories of the Sages that he quotes.

Sforno

Rav Ovadia Sforno (1475-1550) was an Italian commentator. He provides a straightforward explanatory commentary.

Unknown author of Sefer Chinuch (The Book of Education)

This book is a thirteenth century Spanish work of unknown authorship. The author states in his introduction that his goal is to show his young teenage son and his friends that each commandment has a purpose.

Bibliography

Blackman, Philip, F.C.S. *Mishna*. Judaica Press, Ltd., Gateshead, 1977.

Chasida, Yisrael Yitzchak. *Ishei Hatanach BaAspaklaria shel Chazal*. Reuven Mass, Jerusalem, 1988.

Faber, Adele and Elaine Mazlish. *Siblings Without Rivalry*. W.W. Norton and Company, New York, 1987.

Hirsch, Samson Raphael. *Pentateuch Translation and Commentary. Genesis, Exodus, Deuteronomy* volumes. Judaica Press, Gateshead, 1999.

Kranc, Moshe. *The Hasidic Masters' Guide to Management*. Devora Publishing, Jerusalem, 2004.

Leibowitz, Nehama. *Studies in Bereshit (Genesis)*. Hebrew edition, Eliner Library, Joint Authority for Jewish Zionist Education, Dept. for Torah Education and Culture in the Diaspora, Jerusalem.

Maimonides, Moses (Rambam), translator M. Friedlander. *Guide for the Perplexed*. Dover Publications, Inc., New York, 1956.

Maimonides, Moses. *Yad Chazaka*.

Maimonides, Moses. *Letter on Astrology*.

Pelcovitz, Rabbi Raphael. *Sforno: Commentary on the Torah*, Artscroll Mesorah Series. Mesorah Publications, Ltd., 2001, Brooklyn, NY.

Seligman, Martin E. P., Karen Reivich, Lisa Jaycox, Jane Gillham. *The Optimistic Child: Proven Program to Safeguard Children from Depression & Build Lifelong Resistance.* Houghton Mifflin Company, Boston/New York, 1995.

Soloveitchik, Rabbi Joseph B. *Fate and Destiny: From Holocaust to the State of Israel.* Ktav Publishing House, Inc., Hoboken, 2000.